THEORETICAL LINGUISTICS AND DISORDERED LANGUAGE

Edited by Martin J. Ball, Department of Behavioural and Communication Studies, The Polytechnic of Wales

The rapid increase of interest in disordered speech and language among linguists over the past decade or so has resulted in many books of practical help to speech pathologists in terms of assessment and remediation. Little, however, has appeared to examine the theoretical implications of the inter-action between these two fields. This book aims to fill this gap, by showing how speech pathology can inform linguistic theory and vice versa. It is written at the level of the senior student or researcher by leading workers from the UK and USA and should represent a major advance for linguists and speech pathologists.

THEORETICAL LINGUISTICS
AND DISORDERED LANGUAGE

Edited by
MARTIN J. BALL

CROOM HELM
London & Sydney

© 1988 Martin J. Ball
Croom Helm Ltd, 11 New Fetter Lane,
London EC4P 4EE
Croom Helm Australia, 44-50 Waterloo Road,
North Ryde, 2113, New South Wales

British Library Cataloguing in Publication Data

Theoretical linguistics and disordered
    language.
    1. Language disorders   2. Linguistics
    I. Ball, Martin J.
    616.85'5   RC423

    ISBN 0-7099-5012-8

Printed and bound in Great Britain by
St Edmundsbury Press Ltd, Bury St. Edmunds, Suffolk

To my Mother

Contents

Contributors

Martin J. Ball
Senior Lecturer in Linguistics, Department of Behavioural and Communication Studies, Polytechnic of Wales, UK

Shula Chiat
Lecturer in Linguistics, Department of Clinical Communication Studies, City University, London, UK

Chris Code
Senior Lecturer in Neurolinguistics and Neuropsychology, School of Speech Pathology, Leicester Polytechnic, UK

John H. Connolly
Lecturer in Artificial Intelligence, Department of Computer Studies, Loughborough University, UK

Martin Duckworth
Senior Lecturer in Linguistics and Phonetics, School of Speech Therapy, South Glamorgan Institute of Higher Education, UK

Victoria A. Fromkin
Professor of Linguistics, Dean of the Graduate Division, University of California, Los Angeles, USA

Yosef Grodzinsky
Tel Aviv University, Israel, and Boston University School of Medicine, USA

Eirian V. Jones
Department of Speech Therapy, Addenbrooke's Hospital, Cambridge, UK

Niklas Miller
Department of Speech Therapy, Frenchay Hospital, Bristol, UK

Robert S. Pierce
Professor, School of Speech Pathology and Audiology, Kent State University, USA

Rae Smith   Senior Lecturer in Speech Pathology,
School of Speech Pathology, Leicester
Polytechnic, UK

Andrew Spencer   Département de langue et littérature
anglaises, Université de Genève,
22 Boulevard des Philosophes, CH-1205,
Genève, Switzerland

Acknowledgements

I would like to thank those who helped during the preparation of this book: Chris Code for many valuable discussions which helped decide the final shape of the book, and Chrissie Code for putting up with us during all these discussions. Also, for their valuable moral support: Nicole Müller, Pam Harris, Peter Loschi, Georgina Smith and the Arktarians.

Preface

Clinical linguistics has come a long way over the past fifteen years or so, and its tentative beginnings have developed into a recognised area of interdisciplinary study. Initially, perhaps, linguists saw this area as a one-way process: the contribution of linguistics to the description and analysis of disordered language. However, more recently clinical linguistics has seen the initiation of work investigating the contribution of disordered language data to developments in theoretical linguistics.

This book is an attempt to take further these developing links between the theoretical aspects of linguistics on the one hand, and the application of that theory to disordered language on the other. It is, moreover, a deliberate intention of this collection to promote the two-way process already mentioned: to explore not only how theoretical linguistics can inform our study of the non-normal, but how that very study can inform our theory-building.

A collection of work that aims to join these two areas of investigation will need to cover not only as many areas of theoretical linguistics as possible, but also as many areas of clinical language study. In this collection I have attempted, within the space available, to ensure that these major areas have been tackled, though naturally it is not exhaustive in its coverage. The major criterion used for the inclusion of an area of study was its centrality to the concerns of either theoretical or clinical linguistics, even if this meant that some areas of interest had to be excluded.

This book addresses most of the core concerns of theoretical linguistics: phonetics, both descriptive and in terms of models of speech production; phonology, in particular recent trends in non-segmental phonology, and models of phonological acquisition; syntax, especially the development of government-binding theory; semantics and the examination of context. Further areas of linguistic interest include the work reported here on psycholinguistics, pragmatics and bilingualism.

On the other hand, the book includes work on many of the important areas of clinical linguistics and speech pathology. Several of the chapters include discussion on adult-acquired disorders such as aphasia, and apraxia of speech. A range of organic speech disorders are noted in the chapter on phonetic description, and the problems of developmental speech and language disorders are featured in many of the contributions. A major survey of linguistics and stuttering represents a step forward in the clinical linguistic investigation of disorders of fluency. Also included is a chapter on clinical assessment techniques, and the contribution to this area of linguistic theory.

While no collection of studies in a still-developing field of investigation can claim to be complete, I feel that this collection, written by experts in their respective topics, does take the still new area of clinical linguistics a step forward. The book demonstrates that in this interdisciplinary field, not only can theory aid application, but the practice of linguistics with disordered language can tell us something about how to build our theories.

M.J.B.

Foreword

Victoria A. Fromkin
University of California, Los Angeles

In the 5th century BCE, the Greco-Roman physicians recognised that the loss of speech and language was often associated with paralysis of the right side of the body. But it wasn't until Broca presented his seminal paper in Paris in 1861 that this phenomenon was related to the left side of the brain. Almost one hundred years had to pass before such language breakdown was shown to have a bearing on linguistic theory, when, in 1940, Roman Jacobson's *Kindersprache, Aphasie und allgemeine Lautgesetze* was published. However, research on how a study of language disorders can provide insights into normal language (and vice versa) did not really gain a large number of adherents until the 1970s.

This volume, containing eleven chapters concerned with the relationship between linguistic theory and various language disorders shows that the legitimacy of this question is now assumed. The growing interdisciplinary research among, for example, linguists, speech pathologists, neuropsychologists, neurologists, and aphasiologists is producing answers to questions about the brain/mind/language relationship that may, in time, lead to a real understanding of the biology of language.

One may ask why linguists who are concerned with developing a theory of human language and grammar (the cognitive system that represents speakers' knowledge of language) should be interested in disordered language. It is a long held view in the life sciences, that one may learn something about the functioning of a normal system by investigating what results when a breakdown of a part of that system occurs. This has proved to be the case in studying language disorders with the converging evidence that focal damage to the left cerebral hemisphere does not necessarily lead to a total breakdown of language or language processing. Furthermore, since Wernicke pointed out that a lesion in a different area of the left temporal lobe than that sustained by Broca's patient results in a different form of language disorder, there is recognition that lesions to different parts of the left brain effect language and language processing selectively and in a remarkably consistent fashion. For linguistic theory, what is important, is that the parts of the linguistic system which seem to be independently impaired, parallel the modules or components of the grammar that have been proposed by linguistics to account for normal language and language use.

Data collected from patients with language disorders are therefore providing additional evidence in the testing of linguistic theory, and are proving to be crucial in the attempt to uncover or discover the genetic basis for human acquisition and use of language. In addition such research is revealing how language is independent of other cognitive systems since language can be disordered with other cognitive abilities remaining intact, or vice versa. It also shows how language and language use (speech and comprehension) may diverge, in that one may retain knowledge of language but have difficulty in accessing that knowledge; if, for example, a patient produces a jargon version of a word at one time, but a correct pronunciation at another time, clearly this is an access difficulty rather than a representation loss.

The application of linguistic theory to the study of language disorders, and even to the development of new clinical therapy techniques is also having a profound effect. It was once commonplace for clinicians in attempting to diagnose and/or treat patients with language or speech disorders to be rather naive about the nature and structure of language. Linguistic ability was too often equated with the ability to name objects or produce on demand a list of words beginning with a particular 'letter'. Without knowledge of the phonological, syntactic, and semantic complexities of the particular language of the patients, the analysis of their spontaneous speech when asked to describe a picture could at best be intuitive and overly general rather than specific as to details of the disorder. Speech pathologists have been aware for some time that the ability to distinguish between central language disorders and peripheral articulation difficulties depends on recognition of the distinction between the more abstract phonological system and the articulatory neuro-motor realization of this system in the physical phonetic output. It is more recent that clinical aphasiologists have begun to draw upon knowledge of the complexities of syntactic structures in the diagnosis of speech disorders.

The contents of this volume show how far we have come in the utilization of linguistic concepts in these areas. Agrammatism is no longer viewed as simply 'telegraphic' speech with the loss of 'closed class' morphemes or 'functor words'. The importance of thematic roles, and movement transformations in the analysis of agrammatism is now recognised. The role of phonetic theory in speech pathology is pervasive. The modular concept of grammar provides a framework for investigating phonetic, phonemic, syntactic, semantic, lexical, and pragmatic breakdowns independent of each other.

This volume provides additional evidence for the symbiotic relationship between theoretical linguistics and disordered language. It thus constitutes a contribution to our understanding of both.

1

Language Processing and the Effects of Context in Aphasia

Robert S. Pierce

Over the past 15 years, psycholinguistic research has demon-strated the importance of contextual information in the compre-hension process for both spoken (Flores d'Arcais, 1978) and printed information (Rumelhart, 1977). More recently, the role of context in the comprehension process of aphasic adults has been studied. This chapter reviews some of the concepts that have emerged from the normal literature and discusses how context influences aphasic patients' comprehension.

INTERACTIVE PROCESSING IN NORMALS

Issues central to psycholinguistic research are what sources of information are used during word recognition and when they are used. Sources of information include the acoustic–phonetic signal (bottom-up processing) and contextual information (top-down processing). The context consists of semantic, syntactic and pragmatic information that is based on the listener's world knowledge and the constraints of the immediate linguistic/ extralinguistic environments.

Several theories of word recognition exist. However, they differ as to how the information sources interact to activate the mental representation of the word. The logogen theory (Morton, 1969, 1979, 1982) claims that a 'word' in the mental lexicon is represented by a logogen which contains all of the relevant semantic, syntactic, phonologic and orthographic infor-mation about that word. The logogen is a passive device which monitors information from the acoustic–phonetic signal and from the context. When sufficient information is obtained from either source, or from both sources combined, the logogen's threshold is achieved and the word becomes activated. The important aspect of this theory is that information from the acoustic–phonetic signal and from the context is able to activate the logogen. It does not really matter where the information comes from as long as threshold is reached. Thus, the logogen theory is a highly interactive model which allows the listener (or reader) to obtain information from wherever s/he can to aid in identifying words.

In contrast, the cohort theory (Marslen-Wilson, 1975; Marslen-Wilson and Welsh, 1978; Marslen-Wilson and Tyler, 1980) states that there are two stages to word recognition. In the first stage the initial portion of the acoustic–phonetic signal activates a cohort of words that is consistent with the acoustic–phonetic structure. In the second stage the additional acoustic–phonetic signal and/or the context acts on the cohort to reduce it to a single appropriate word. Accordingly, the acoustic–phonetic signal plays an important role initially in developing the cohort of word possibilities. Context plays a subsequent role in helping to select a word from the cohort.

Several researchers have taken issue with the notion that only the acoustic–phonetic signal is able to generate a cohort of word possibilities. Grosjean (1980), using a gating procedure, suggested that both acoustic–phonetic and contextual sources of information are able to generate a cohort of word possibilities. More recently, Salasoo and Pisoni (1985) demonstrated that while word identification is most efficient when phonetic–acoustic information and normal sentential constraints are present, word identification is possible without acoustic–phonetic information from the beginning of words. An interaction between the two sources of information was also demonstrated. Salasoo and Pisoni found that as more acoustic–phonetic information became available, the influence of the contextual information decreased. This research suggests that both the acoustic–phonetic signal and context are active in the initial stages of word identification, which is consistent with Morton's logogen theory.

Unlike the logogen and the cohort models which allow for interaction between bottom-up and top-down sources of information, Forster's (1976, 1979) theory is strictly bottom-up in nature. The acoustic–phonetic signal activates an entry in a peripheral access file which then locates an entry in the master lexicon. This information is then passed on to a syntactic processor and finally to a message processor. This theory is serial in nature, stating that information flows in one direction and that lexical access is not influenced by higher levels. Contextual information interacts with the information received from the bottom-up sources at the level of the message processor in order to determine the meaning of the utterance. Support for this theory comes from Cairns, Cowart and Jablon (1981). It is also consistent with studies (e.g. Swinney, 1979) showing that context does not initially restrict the activation of different meanings of ambiguous words. Rather, context plays a role in selecting the one appropriate meaning at a later time, such as at the end of clauses (vanDijk and Kintsch, 1983).

An aspect of contextual influence that has been studied more recently relates to the differential strength of contextual environments. In general, this notion has been studied by using sentential contexts that vary in the degree to which they predict a particular word (Bloom and Fischler, 1980). For example, Simpson (1981) reported that when an ambiguous word appeared in a highly constraining sentence (i.e. one that strongly predicted one particular meaning of the word), only the contextually consistent meaning was retrieved. Schwanenflugel and Shoben (1985) used a lexical decision paradigm to study the effects of high and low constraining sentences on the facilitation of expected and unexpected words. They found a narrow scope of facilitation for the highly constraining sentences that facilitated the expected word but inhibited the unexpected word. In contrast, the low constraining sentences generated a broader, weaker facilitation that effected both expected and unexpected words.

While the degree of contextual facilitation varies as a function of characteristics of the context, it also depends on characteristics of the listener. Daneman and Green (1986) demonstrated that the ability to use context to help in the comprehension process related to the individual's working memory capacity. Working memory was measured with a test that taxes both the processing and storage functions of working memory during sentence comprehension. Those subjects with smaller working memories were less able to use context to determine meanings for unusual words than were those with larger working memories. The authors theorised that those individuals with smaller working memories devote a greater

3

percentage of their capacity to the reading process, and have less residual capacity for retaining the relevant contextual cues.

This brief review clearly does not do justice to the complexity of the issues involved. However, it serves to point out that comprehension is a highly interactive process, and that context is intimately involved at several stages of the process. Specifically, context aids in word identification and in determining a meaning for the message. Context varies in the degree to which it is useful and some individuals are better at using context than are others.

There is an interaction between the need to process the acoustic–phonetic and the contextual information that depends on the situation. For example, in the sentence 'I went to the store and bought a ring.', the listener would need to hear most of the word ring before recognising it. However, in 'I went to the jewellery store and bought a ring.', less of the acoustic–phonetic information associated with ring would need to be processed before recognition occurred. In the narrative 'I am getting married next month. I need to go to a jewelry store and pick out a ring for my bride.', it is questionable whether any of the acoustic–phonetic signal associated with ring would need to be processed in order for the word to be mentally accessed.

Context does not need to be linguistically based. The sentence 'What do you mean you forgot the ...' would require the listener to rely on the acoustic–phonetic information in order to understand the last word (tickets, beer, keys, kids, etc.). However, when the sentence is exclaimed by a man dressed in white standing at a church altar to his soon-to-be-ex best man, no additional acoustic–phonetic information is really needed. This is similar to the contextual facilitation generated by scripts (Sharkey and Mitchell, 1985) and underscores the importance of world knowledge to the comprehension process. The remainder of this chapter will examine how aphasic individuals use context during language processing.

CONTEXTUAL INFLUENCES ON COMPREHENSION IN APHASIA

It is well established that aphasic individuals have varying degrees of difficulty processing syntactic and semantic information. This section explores the effect of placing specific syntactic and semantic processing demands within a contextual environment. Issues to be discussed include contextual influences on non-literal versus literal meanings, influence of world knowledge and linguistic/extralinguistic environments as contextual sources, and interaction between contextual and acoustic–phonetic sources of information.

Non-literal meanings

Non-literal expressions carry a special role in language because they require the listener to construct a meaning that is typically different from the meaning associated with the words themselves. These include such expressions as metaphors, idioms and indirect requests. For example, the sentence 'They shot the bull.' has a very different meaning in reference to two men with guns on a farm compared to two men sitting around a fireplace talking. The question is whether aphasic individuals can recognize the non-literal meaning of the expression when it is provided in an appropriate context.

Stachowiak, Huber, Poeck and Kerschensteiner (1977) presented aphasic subjects with narratives that contained metaphoric expressions and asked them to select a picture to indicate what happened; see (1).

(1) Werner and his wife meet with friends every Friday. This time the men want to play poker. Because Werner plays riskily, he soon loses all of his money. The others strip him right down to his shirt. His wife gets quite annoyed. Which picture shows what happened to him?

They found that the aphasic subjects performed as well as did the normals, and suggested that the redundancy of the narrative compensates for the difficulties aphasic individuals have in comprehending isolated words and sentences.

Myers and Linebaugh (1981) noted that the third sentence in Stachowiak *et al.*'s narratives provided a literal interpretation of the target information and that the metaphor served primarily to amplify or reiterate the information. To reduce the redundancy and test for comprehension of the metaphor, Myers and Linebaugh presented narratives such as (2).

(2) Jim knew that the office accounts were wrong by about 1000 dollars because of mistakes he had made. For weeks he hesitated to show the account books to the boss, but finally he decided he had to go in and just face the music.

They found that their aphasic subjects also performed as well as did the normals, suggesting that aphasic individuals are able to determine the non-literal meaning of metaphors and idioms in context.

The ability of aphasic subjects to understand indirect requests was studied by Wilcox, Davis and Leonard (1978). They presented aphasic subjects with videotaped vignettes of a person making an indirect request of another person in an appropriate situation (e.g. a person holding a lot of books asking another person 'Can you open the door?'). The aphasic subjects viewed the tapes and indicated whether the second person's response was appropriate or not. The authors found that the aphasic subjects performed better than their scores on standardized language tests would have suggested. These studies suggest that aphasic individuals are able to appreciate the non-literal meaning of utterances when they are presented within appropriate contexts.

Literal meanings

Unlike non-literal meanings, literal meanings convey essentially the same information whether presented in isolation or in context. Since aphasic individuals are impaired at understanding much of this information, the main issue is whether context helps them understand the conveyed meaning better than if no context existed. The target information can be either semantically or syntactically based and the context can relate to world knowledge, the linguistic/extralinguistic environment, and/or paralinguistic information.

World knowledge

A person's knowledge of how the world works, i.e. reality, can influence how s/he interprets information. Several studies have demonstrated that aphasic individuals are sensitive to the use of world knowledge and understand messages better when they can use reality to guide their processing. For example, reversible active sentences such as 'The girl charms the soldier' require the listener to undertake a syntactic analysis to determine the subject/object relationship. However, Deloche and Seron (1981) demonstrated that aphasics subjects' comprehension improves if one of the subject/object relationships is more plausible than the other based on reality (e.g. 'The lion devours the antelope'). This was true for Broca's aphasic subjects but not for subjects with Wernicke's aphasia. A way to conceptualise this distinction is simply to list the key lexical items in each sentence, as in (3a) and (3b).

(3a) girl	(3b) lion
charms	devours
soldier	antelope

Lists such as (3b), which can be ordered based on a semantic/pragmatic strategy, are easier to understand than lists that are not able to be so ordered. Aphasics can supplement their impaired syntactic processing skills with this type of semantic/pragmatic strategy.

Kudo (1984) expanded on this finding. He tested the comprehension of plausible versus implausible sentences and found that the plausible sentences were comprehended more accurately than were the implausible sentences by subjects with Broca's, Wernicke's, amnesic and global aphasia. This difference was evident for both syntactic contrasts (e.g. 'A dog chases a cat.' versus 'A girl bites a dog.') and lexical contrasts (e.g. 'A girl has a pencil.' versus 'A man throws a car.'). In addition, syntactic items were comprehended more accurately when a plausible item (e.g. 'A dog bites a girl.') was placed in competition with a non-plausible foil (e.g. 'A girl bites a dog.') than when both foils were plausible (e.g. 'A dog chases a cat.' and 'A cat chases a dog.') In the first instance the subjects could use a semantic strategy to determine the subject/object relationship while in the second instance they could not.

World knowledge also influences the appreciation of locative prepositions (Seron and Deloche, 1981). When asked to place a movable object in/on/under a non-movable object, subjects with Broca's aphasia were more accurate when the requested relationship was consistent with the objects' normal relationship than when it was not. For example, *under* was comprehended

7

more accurately than *on* for the request 'Put the shoes under/ on the bed.'. However, *on* was easier than *under* for the request 'Put the soap on/under the hand basin.'.

The extreme case of plausibility based on world knowledge consists of non-reversible sentences. These sentences, such as reversible passives, depict semantic relationships that have only one logical interpretation (e.g. 'The flower was picked by the girl.' and 'The apple that the boy is eating is red.'). That these non-reversible sentences are much easier for aphasic subjects to understand than are reversible sentences is well established (Caramazza and Zurif, 1976; Heilman, Scholes and Watson, 1976; Kolk and Friederici, 1985; Pierce and Wagner, 1985).

The ability to apply world knowledge to the comprehension process implies that the relevant knowledge is intact. Certain types of knowledge may be more available to aphasic individuals than others. Wallace and Canter (1985) reported that aphasic subjects understood spoken and printed personal questions better than non-personal questions. Gray, Hoyt, Mogil and Lefkowitz (1977) found that the general information yes/no questions from the *Western Aphasia Battery* (Kertesz, 1982) were more difficult for aphasic subjects than were the enviromental and personal questions. Information with a strong emotional component is often processed better by aphasic subjects than is non-emotional information (Boller, Cole, Vrtunski, Patterson and Kim, 1979; Landis, Graves and Goodglass, 1982).

This research indicates that aphasic individuals can use their world knowledge to facilitate comprehension. Accuracy improves when they can supplement an impaired processing system with a strategy based on the pragmatics of world knowledge.

Linguistic/extralinguistic context

The research examining the influence of linguistic/extralinguistic context on comprehension has used two distinct paradigms. In the first, comprehension of target information has been assessed with and without specific context. Since the aphasic subjects usually indicated comprehension by pointing to pictures or answering questions, the integration of the target information and the context could occur late in the comprehension process, such as at the level of a message processor. In most instances, comprehension has been better when some form of context was present than when it was not.

Waller and Darley (1978) compared aphasic subjects' comprehension of paragraphs that were either presented alone or preceded by short verbal prestimulations. For example, one paragraph was preceded by the context 'This story is about a man named Charles Fredericks, who wanted to cross Antarctica. At that time no one had yet done it. Antarctica was a cold and barren continent.' (p. 744). The authors found that cohesive paragraphs were comprehended more accurately with the contextual sentences than without. In a subsequent report, Waller and Darley (1979) tested the comprehension of individual sentences, containing a variety of syntactic structures, both with and without preceding contextual sentences. In this case the aphasic subjects' comprehension was equivalent for both conditions. Two possible reasons for this lack of contextual facilitation were suggested by the authors. One, the subjects were functioning at a fairly high level. Their average score in the acontextual condition was 76 per cent so a ceiling effect may have been operative. Two, the contextual sentences were rather general in nature and may not have provided sufficient information to influence the plausibility of the relationships contained in the target sentences. Further research has helped to clarify these issues.

Pierce and Wagner (1985) tested aphasic subjects' comprehension of reversible passive sentences in three conditions. One, the passive sentence was presented in isolation. Two, the passive sentence was preceded by a sentence that did not predict the subject/object relationship in the target sentence, as in (4a). Three, the passive sentence was preceded by a sentence that did predict the appropriate subject/object relationship, as in (4b).

(4a) The boy and girl are playing.
     The boy is carried by the girl.
     Who is carried?

(4b) The boy sprained his ankle.
     The boy is carried by the girl.
     Who is carried?

The subjects achieved significantly higher scores when the predictive contextual sentence was present than when the passive sentence was presented in isolation. The non-predictive contextual sentence condition did not generate a significant improvement compared to the isolation condition. The operative mechanism is probably similar to the influence of world knowledge reviewed previously. The predictive contextual sentence generates an environment where the passive sentence is no longer freely reversible. One subject/object relationship becomes more plausible than the other so the aphasic subjects can use this semantic/pragmatic strategy in lieu of a strictly syntactic analysis. The non-predictive context sentence did not significantly improve comprehension because it did not impact on the plausibility of the forthcoming subject/object relationship. Pierce and Wagner divided their subjects into high and low comprehension groups. The results discussed above were evident only for the low comprehension group. The high comprehension group did not significantly benefit from the contextual conditions, which is consistent with Waller and Darley (1979).

Pierce and Beekman (1985) expanded on these results by using syntactic and semantic target information as well as linguistic and extralinguistic context. They tested reversible passives and active declaratives (e.g. 'The girl was peeling an onion.') in three conditions: (a) isolation, (b) preceded by a predictive sentence, as in (5), and (c) preceded by a picture that depicted the same information as contained in the predictive contextual sentence.

(5) The girl was crying.
The girl was peeling an onion (banana).
What was she peeling?

The subjects achieved significantly higher scores in both the linguistic (sentences) and extralinguistic (pictures) contextual conditions than in the isolation condition. Again, these results were evident only for the low comprehension group. When the environment establishes a situation where certain events are more likely to occur, aphasic individuals seem able to use that knowledge to improve their comprehension efficiency.

It is not necessary for the contextual information to precede the target information. Pierce (1986) demonstrated that contextual sentences were equally beneficial whether they occurred prior to the target information, as in (6a), or following it, as in (6b).

(6a) The teacher has a black eye.
The teacher was hit by the boy.
Who was hit?

(6b) The girl was pulled by the boy.
The girl was sitting in a wagon.
Who was pulled?

The same result was found for both syntactic and semantic target information. Aphasic individuals can integrate contextual and target information, regardless of order of presentation, as long as both sources of information occur prior to the need to respond. This pattern is consistent with integration at the level of a message processor (Cairns *et al.*, 1981).

The preceding research suggests that the contextual information must be semantically or pragmatically predictive in order to be effective. However, Cannito, Jarecki and Pierce (1986) demonstrated contextual facilitation using narratives that were non-predictive. They assessed aphasic subjects' comprehension of reversible active and passive sentences presented in isolation and when preceded by five-sentence narratives that, by design, did not predict one or the other subject/object relationship. Comprehension was significantly better when the active and passive sentences were preceded by the narratives than when they were presented in isolation. This result suggests that aphasic listeners may benefit from a redundancy in what they hear. After hearing the same topic nouns throughout the narratives, the listener may be able to devote more processing attention to the relationship between the nouns as depicted in the final target sentences. When the target sentence is presented in isolation, processing attention must be divided between understanding the meaning of the nouns and determining the relationship between them.

Hough, Pierce and Cannito (1986) further analysed this issue by assessing the comprehension of reversible passives in isolation and following five-sentence narratives that either did or did not predict the target subject/object relationship. They found two distinct patterns. Some of the aphasic subjects benefited from the narrative context regardless of whether or not it predicted the target relationship. Other subjects benefited only from the predictive narratives. Both contextual conditions can be beneficial, but their use varies across subjects and may relate to individual characteristics of the listener (Daneman and Green, 1986).

The second paradigm used to evaluate contextual influences in aphasic listeners is a word monitoring task. In this task, subjects are presented a sentence and asked to indicate when they hear a previously specified word. The extent to which the target word is predictable based on semantic, syntactic and/or pragmatic information in the sentence is varied, and the effect of this variation on the subject's response latency is used as a measure of contextual influence. Several studies (Friederici, 1983, 1985; Tyler, 1985) have shown that aphasic subjects were sensitive to semantic and pragmatic constraints during on-line processing. That is, their response latencies became significantly shorter when the target word was predicted by the semantic constraints of the sentence. They were less sensitive to syntactic constraints. These results indicate that aphasic individuals can use linguistic contextual information to supplement the information derived from the acoustic–phonetic signal. When contextual constraints are strong, less acoustic–phonetic information is needed in order to make lexical decisions.

The interaction of contextual and acoustic–phonetic information was also evaluated by Beck (1984) and Pierce and DeStefano (in press). Beck asked aphasic subjects to indicate which of two phonemically similar words they heard in sentences (e.g. state/steak). Accuracy was greatest when the sentence was congruent ('The state was Wisconsin'). The subjects were less accurate when the sentence was neutral ('The state was included'), and least accurate when it was incongruent ('The state was sirloin').

Pierce and DeStefano (1987) tested the comprehension of target nouns contained in the middle of three-sentence narratives. In half of the stimuli the entire acoustic–phonetic signal for the target word was presented. In the other half only the initial sound sequence was presented. The narratives were divided into three levels based on the degree to which they predicted the target word. The results indicated that as the narratives became more predictive of the target word, the subjects relied less on the acoustic–phonetic signal and more on the contextual information for comprehension. In the strong predictive narrative, comprehension accuracy was equivalent for both levels of acoustic signal integrity. These results indicate that aphasic individuals can use contextual information to supplement what they obtain from the acoustic signal, especially if the acoustic signal (or their perception of it) is degraded.

The research reviewed in this section demonstrates that aphasic individuals use linguistic/extralinguistic context during several aspects of the comprehension process. They can use context to supplement information derived from the acoustic signal during word identification. They can also use context to enrich their understanding of words contained in a message.

Paralinguistic influences

Several studies have shown that aphasic individuals can use paralinguistic features such as prosody to assist in comprehension. Green and Boller (1974) demonstrated that severely impaired aphasic subjects recognised whether an utterance was a statement, question or a command although they failed to appreciate the linguistic content of the message. Blumstein and Goodglass (1972) reported that aphasic subjects used syllabic stress and juncture to differentiate between words that had the same phonetic construction (e.g. 'convict': noun versus verb; 'sorehead' versus 'sore head'). Baum, Daniloff, Daniloff and Lewis (1982) also demonstrated that aphasic subjects retained some ability to use stress and juncture to disambiguate sentences, even though their performance was significantly worse than normals.

Pashek and Brookshire (1982) conducted a direct test of the influence of stress on comprehension. They assessed aphasic subjects' comprehension of information contained in paragraphs presented (1) with a normal stress pattern and (2) with emphasised stress on crucial words throughout the paragraph. They found significantly better comprehension with the emphasised stress than with the normal stress pattern.

CLINICAL IMPLICATIONS

The clinical implications of this research are two-fold. First, it is important to recognise what sources of information a patient can use during any particular diagnostic or treatment task. For example, Nicholas, MacLennan and Brookshire (1986) administered the reading comprehension subtests from several standard aphasia batteries by giving the questions without the stimulus texts. Two such questions, from the *Boston Diagnostic*

13

Aphasia Examination (Goodglass and Kaplan, 1983), are 'Another kind of artist is a ... picture ... musician ... library ... soldier' and 'Sterilization by heat is a result of ... sanitation ... good food ... Pasteur's discovery ... germs'. The authors found that over half of the questions were consistently responded to correctly. This suggests that aphasic patients can apply world knowledge to this comprehension task, and that their performance may not be a valid measure of their 'paragraph' comprehension skills. A similar distinction can be found in popular clinical workbooks where some of the questions used for paragraph comprehension tasks require extracting information from the paragraph while others do not. It is important for clinicians to recognise this distinction and use it to determine levels of difficulty of their stimulus items.

The patient's ability to understand specific information within a paragraph will also be influenced by the extent to which that information is predicted by the linguistic context. For example, the stimulus item in (7a) will be easier than (7b) because the target information is more highly constrained by the paragraph.

(7a) The sky looks very cloudy today.
      Perhaps you should take your umbrella.
      It is supposed to rain all day.
      What should you take today?

(7b) The children went to the zoo.
      One child had never seen a zebra.
      He talked about the trip for weeks.
      What had the child not seen before?

A computerised treatment program developed at Kent State University maintains separate scores based on this distinction, and patients consistently perform better in the highly predictive paragraphs than on the less predictive ones.

Similar influences are evident at the sentence level. For example, the stimulus sentence 'I went to the (hardware) store and bought some nails. What did I buy?' would be easier with 'hardware' included because it limits the numbers of items that could be bought.

Aphasic patients' ability to use extralinguistic context has dramatic implications for treatment. It may be that a patient's inability to understand an utterance during a contextually barren treatment session does not reflect his/her inability to understand that utterance in an appropriate contextual environment. A patient may not understand simple commands during the speech therapy treatment session, yet may follow similar commands accurately during a physical therapy session. The nature of the physical therapist's commands is often supported by the extralinguistic context. Similarly, a patient may have difficulty pointing to 'salt' from an array of pictures, yet readily find it at the dinner table when asked to pass it. This distinction may also contribute to the notion that spouses often feel aphasic patients communicate better than the clinicians feel they do (Helmick, Watamori and Palmer, 1976).

The second implication is that the traditional hierarchy of difficulty of word–sentence–paragraph loses some validity. Information contained in sentences becomes easier to understand if other sentences are presented with it that semantically and pragmatically support that information (Pierce and Wagner, 1985; Pierce and Beekman, 1985). Although not yet systematically studied, it may be that the comprehension of single words would be easier in a supportive context. For example, Pierce (1984) demonstrated that aphasic subjects were more accurate in identifying typical meanings of homographs than less typical meanings (e.g. 'to hit' versus 'worn out' for the homograph 'beat'). It is conceivable that the less typical meaning would be better appreciated if heard from an exhausted housewife who said 'I cooked and cleaned house all day. I am beat.' than if presented in isolation in a treatment room. Clinicians should be aware that, depending on the particular stimuli, single word level tasks are not necessarily easier than sentence level tasks which may be more difficult than paragraph level tasks.

SUMMARY

In a manner similar to normals, aphasic individuals use contextual information to assist in language processing. They can use context interactively with the acoustic–phonetic signal to assist in word identification. They can use context at later stages of processing to strengthen their understanding of the message. Aphasic individuals can derive contextual information from their world knowledge and from the linguistic/extralinguistic environment. Recognition of the role of context in language processing impacts on diagnostic and treatment procedures. Future endeavours with aphasic patients will need to reflect these influences.

NOTE

1. Several studies have shown that aphasic subjects have auditory perceptual/discrimination problems (Basso, Casati and Vignolo, 1977; Miceli, Gainotti, Caltagirone and Masullo, 1980). However, a typical finding has been that many of those subjects with perceptual problems also have good comprehension skills. This paradox led Miceli *et al.* (1980) to state what 'other factors such as contextual cues, previous language knowledge, acoustic and semantic constraints may provide additional pieces of information needed for the correct understanding of the verbal auditory input even when some steps are defective' (p. 168).

REFERENCES

Basso, A., Casati, B. and Vignolo, L. (1977) Phonemic identification defect in aphasia. *Cortex, 13*, 84-95

Baum, S., Daniloff, J., Daniloff, R. and Lewis, J. (1982) Sentence comprehension by Broca's aphasics: effects of some supragegmental variables. *Brain and Language, 17*, 261-71

Beck, A. (1984) The processing of the sounds and meanings of ongoing speech by aphasic subjects. *Brain and Language, 22*, 320-38

Bloom, P. and Fischler, I. (1980) Completion norms for 329 sentence contexts. *Memory and Cognition, 8*, 631-42

Blumstein, S. and Goodglass, H. (1972) The perception of stress as a semantic cue in aphasia. *Journal of Speech and Hearing Research, 15*, 800-6

Boller, F., Cole, M., Vrtunski, B., Patterson, M. and Kim, Y. (1979) Paralinguistic aspects of auditory comprehension in aphasia. *Brain and Language, 7*, 164-74

Cairns, H., Cowart, W. and Jablon, A. (1981) Effect of prior context upon the integration of lexical information during sentence processing. *Journal of Verbal Learning and Verbal Behavior, 20*, 445-53

Cannito, M., Jarecki, J. and Pierce, R. (1986) Effects of thematic structure on syntactic comprehension in aphasia. *Brain and Language, 27*, 38-49

Caramazza, A. and Zurif, E. (1976) Dissociation of algorithmic and heuristic processes in language comprehension: evidence from aphasia. *Brain and Language, 3*, 572-82

Daneman, M. and Green, I. (1986) Individual differences in comprehending and producing words in context. *Journal of Memory and*

Language, 25, 1-18

Deloche, G. and Seron, X. (1981) Sentence understanding and know-ledge of the world: evidence from a sentence–picture matching task performed by aphasic patients. *Brain and Language, 14,* 57-69

vanDijk, T. and Kintsch, W. (1983) *Strategies of discourse comprehension,* Academic Press, New York

Flores d'Arcais, G. (1978) The perception of complex sentences. In Levelt, W. and Flores d'Arcais, G. (eds), *Studies in the perception of language,* Wiley, London

Forster, K. (1976) Accessing the mental lexicon. In Wales, R. and Walker, E. (eds), *New approaches to language mechanism,* North Holland, Amsterdam

Forster, K. (1979) Levels of processing and the structure of the language processor. In Cooper, W. and Walker, E. (eds), *Sentence Processing: Psycholinguistic Studies Presented to Merrill Garrett,* Lawrence Erlbaum Associates, Hillsdale

Friederici, A. (1983) Aphasics' perception of words in sentential context: some real-time processing evidence. *Neuropsychologia, 21,* 351-8

Friederici, A. (1985) Levels of processing and vocabulary types: evidence from on-line comprehension in normals and agrammatics. *Cognition, 19,* 133-66

Goodglass, H. and Kaplan, E. (1983) *The assessment of aphasia and related disorders,* Lea & Febiger, Philadelphia

Gray, L., Hoyt, P., Mogil, S. and Lefkowitz, N. (1977) A comparison of clinical tests of yes/no questions in aphasia. In Brookshire, R. (ed.), *Clincial Aphasiology Conference Proceedings,* BRK, Minneapolis

Green, E. and Boller F. (1974) Features of auditory comprehension in severely impaired aphasics. *Cortex, 10,* 133-45

Grosjean, F. (1980) Spoken word recognition processes and the gating paradigm. *Perception and Psychophysics, 28,* 267-83

Heilman, K., Scholes, R. and Watson, R. (1976) Defects of immediate memory in Broca's and conduction aphasia. *Brain and Language, 3,* 201-8

Helmick, J., Watamori, T. and Palmer, J. (1976) Spouses' understanding of the communication disabilities of aphasic patients. *Journal of Speech and Hearing Disorders, 41,* 238-43

Hough, M., Pierce, R. and Cannito, M. (1986) Effects of pragmatically predictive context on syntactic comprehension in aphasia. Paper presented at the annual convention of the American Speech–Language–Hearing Association, Detroit, November

Kertesz, A. (1982) *The Western Aphasia Battery,* Grune & Stratton, New York

Kolk, H. and Friederici, A. (1985) Strategy and impairment in sentence understanding by Broca's and Wernicke's aphasics. *Cortex, 21,* 47-67

Kudo, T. (1984) The effect of semantic plausibility on sentence comprehension in aphasia. *Brain and Language, 21,* 208-18

Landis, T., Graves, R. and Goodglass, H. (1982) Aphasic reading and

17

writing: possible evidence for right hemisphere participation. *Cortex, 18*, 105-11

Marslen-Wilson, W. (1975) Sentence perception as an interactive parallel process. *Science, 189*, 226-8

Marslen-Wilson, W. and Tyler, L. (1980) The temporal structure of spoken language understanding. *Cognition*, 8, 1-71

Marslen-Wilson, W. and Welsh, A. (1978) Processing interactions and lexical access during word recognition in continuous speech. *Cognitive Psychology, 10*, 29-63

Miceli, G., Gainotti, G., Caltagirone, C. and Masullo, C. (1980) Some aspects of phonological impairment in aphasia. *Brain and Language, 11*, 159-69

Morton, J. (1969) Interaction of information in word recognition. *Psychological Review, 76*, 165-78

Morton, J. (1979) Word recognition. In Morton, J. and Marshall, J. (eds), *Psycholinguistics 2: structures and processes*, MIT Press, Cambridge

Morton, J. (1982) Disintegrating the lexicon: an information processing approach. In Mehler, J., Walker, E. and Garrett, M. (eds), *On mental representation*, Lawrence Erlbaum Associates, Hillsdale

Myers, P. and Linebaugh, C. (1981) Comprehension of idiomatic expressions by right-hemisphere-damaged adults. In Brookshire, R. (ed.), *Clinical Aphasiology Conference Proceedings*, BRK, Minneapolis

Nicholas, L., MacLennan, D. and Brookshire, R. (1986) Validity of multiple-sentence reading comprehension tests for aphasic adults. *Journal of Speech and Hearing Disorders, 51*, 82-7

Pashek, G. and Brookshire, R. (1982) Effects of rate of speech and linguistic stress on auditory paragraph comprehension of aphasic individuals. *Journal of Speech and Hearing Research, 25*, 377-82

Pierce, R. (1984) Comprehending homographs in aphasia. *Brain and Language, 22*, 339-49

Pierce, R. (1986) Effects of prior and subsequent context in aphasia. Paper presented at the annual convention of the American Speech–Language–Hearing Association, Detroit, November

Pierce, R. and Beekman, L. (1985) Effects of linguistic and extralinguistic context on semantic and syntactic processing in aphasia. *Journal of Speech and Hearing Research, 28*, 250-4

Pierce, R. and DeStefano, C. (1987). The interactive nature of auditory comprehension in aphasia. *Journal of Communication Disorders, 20*, 15-24

Pierce, R. and Wagner, C. (1985) The role of context in facilitating syntactic decoding in aphasia. *Journal of Communication Disorders, 18*, 203-14

Rumelhart, D. (1977) Toward an interactive model of reading. In Dornic, S. (ed.), *Attention and performance. VI.* Lawrence Erlbaum Associates, Hillsdale

Salasoo, A. and Pisoni, D. (1985) Interaction of knowledge sources in spoken word identification. *Journal of Memory and Language, 24*, 210-31

Schwanenflugel, P. and Shoben, E. (1985) The influence of sentence constraint on the scope of facilitation for upcoming words. *Journal of Memory and Language, 24*, 232-52

Seron, X. and Deloche, G. (1981) Processing of locatives 'in', 'on', and 'under' by aphasic patients: an analysis of the regression hypothesis. *Brain and Language, 14*, 70-80

Sharkey, N. and Mitchell, D. (1985) Word recognition in a functional context: the use of scripts in reading. *Journal of Memory and Language, 24*, 253-70

Simpson, G. (1981) Meaning dominance and semantic context in the processing of lexical ambiguity. *Journal of Verbal Learning and Verbal Behavior, 20*, 120-36

Stachowiak, F., Huber, W., Poeck, K. and Kerschensteiner, M. (1977) Text comprehension in aphasia. *Brain and Language, 4*, 177-95

Swinney, D. (1979) Lexical access during sentence comprehension: reconsideration of context effects. *Journal of Verbal Learning and Verbal Behaviour, 18*, 645-59

Tyler, L. (1985) Real-time comprehension processes in agrammatism: a case study. *Brain and Language, 26*, 259-75

Wallace, G. and Canter, G. (1985) Effects of personally relevant language materials on the performance of severely aphasic individuals. *Journal of Speech and Hearing Disorders, 50*, 385-90

Waller, M. and Darley, F. (1978) The influence of context on the auditory comprehension of paragraphs by aphasic subjects. *Journal of Speech and Hearing Research, 21*, 732-45

Waller, M. and Darley, F. (1979) Effect of prestimulation on sentence comprehension by aphasic subjects. *Journal of Communication Disorders, 12*, 461-9

Wilcox, M., Davis, G. and Leonard, L. (1978) Aphasics' comprehension of contextually conveyed meaning. *Brain and Language, 6*, 362-377

2

Unifying the Various Language-related Sciences: Aphasic Syndromes and Grammatical Theory

Yosef Grodzinsky

The study of the theory of grammar in its modern incarnation is concerned with the knowledge of language humans possess. Under Chomsky's tutelage, linguists have shifted their interests from languages as collections of sentences to abstract principles that underlie the grammatical systems of the world's languages (see, for instance, Chomsky, 1986). In this conceptual framework, linguists are no longer concerned with the study of observed corpora from English, Swahili and French, but rather in the properties that the grammars of these languages share. These are supposed to be inherent in universal grammar, which is taken, in turn, to be the knowledge we are equipped with when we come to the world, without which we could not acquire our mother tongue so naturally and at such ease.

This conception of language has received much press in the past three decades, and there is no need for it to be reiterated in detail here. What is important here is the context in which language is now studied: instead of writing grammars for many languages, irrespective of the speakers of these, now the linguist is studying the grammatical principles that are mentally represented for humans. This means, of course, that the study of grammatical systems is now the study of psychological systems. Indeed, as Chomsky and his colleagues have put it (Chomsky and Miller, 1963), the language sciences are concerned with three related questions: What is the precise nature of our linguistic knowledge? How does it arise in the individual? How is it put to use? Put this way, linguistics is a part of psychology, some would even say — biology, because the study of psychological functions and the machinery that underlies them is the study of systems supported by the brain.

Knowledge of language and mechanisms that put it to use interest other groups of researchers beside linguists. The point of view of generative linguistics has not been the only angle from which one can approach the language faculty. Neuropsychologists, in particular, have been looking at language in quite a different way (see Goodglass and Kaplan, 1972; Geschwind, 1979, for statements of one dominant approach). It seems to me, however, that adjacent disciplines will gain tremendously if they look into each other's achievements.

In the following pages I am going to explore some issues pertaining to the interaction between theories of grammatical representation — linguistic theories and language deficits. I think that confronting the two raises some very hard questions, yet if we succeed in making sense of these, we are likely to embark on a promising journey. Defining the relation between the neuropsychology of language and the theory of language correctly will have, in my view, many interesting and valuable consequences for both. I will attempt to show how key ideas in each of these two areas will, if followed, lead to a point of convergence.

The study of cognitive deficits is interesting because it enables us to get a glimpse at cognitive mechanisms and at the neural tissue supporting them. This unique perspective is made possible due to the *partial* loss of function. Total loss makes our task impossible, as no clear patterns can be identified. How partial a particular loss is, what exactly the correct description of the pattern of selectivity is, and what the theoretical significance of this description is are the crux of the matter.

It appears that there is now plenty of evidence to suggest that, at least in some aphasic syndromes, the pattern of selectivity is best described along grammatical lines. So there are patients who are capable of handling linguistic materials of some sorts, yet fail on others, where the contrast between the two types of materials is grammatical. If this is the case, then there are aspects of the deficit that cannot be described precisely without reference to grammatical concepts. An example of one such deficit should make my point clear.

It is by no means surprising that the example I chose comes from the study of agrammatism. Linguistically it is by far the most-studied language disturbance. Identified as such at the beginning of this century (Pick, 1913) it has been known to have grammatical patterns of selectivity. Consider the comprehension ability of agrammatic aphasic patients. In the past decade it has become increasingly clear that the deficit characteristic of this syndrome is somehow connected to grammatical variables (Caramazza and Zurif, 1976; Zurif and Caramazza, 1976; Schwartz, Saffran and Marin, 1980; Caplan and Futter, 1986; Grodzinsky, 1985a, 1986; Grodzinsky, Finkelstein, Nicol and Zurif, 1985). Below I will present a summary of recent results of a variety of experiments that tested the comprehension of agrammatic aphasics. Specifically I will examine their syntactic ability through the testing of their ability to assign thematic roles (agent, patient, etc.; see, for example, Jackendoff, 1972) to noun phrases, as attested either by their performance in matching semantically reversible sentences to pictures, where the main foil is always thematic role reversal, or by related tasks (such as acting out, or arrangement of sentence fragments).

In (1)–(3) there are three groups of sentences: (1) contains sentence types where agrammatic aphasics performed above chance on the task described above, thus indicating near-normal comprehension ability; (2) contains cases where comprehension is at chance, suggesting that the patients guess; and (3) has a case where the patients performed below chance, which is a sign of consistent reversal of thematic roles:

above chance – correct
(1) (a) The boy pushed the girl.
    (b) The desk supports the chair.
    (c) The man who pushed the woman was fat.
    (d) Show me the man who pushed the woman.
    (e) It is the monkey who bumped the bear.

at chance – guessing
(2) (a) The girl was pushed by the boy.
    (b) The chair is supported by the desk.
    (c) The man who the woman pushed was fat.
    (d) Show me the man who the woman pushed.
    (e) It is the monkey who the bear bumped.

below chance – reversal
(3) (a) The woman was admired by the man.

How are we to account for this differential performance? A quick look at these contrasts suggests that a linguistic account is unavoidable. The contrast between (1c) and (2c), for instance, is expressible in terms of the grammatical function that the NP *the woman* has in the embedded clause. Moreover, the performance contrast between (2a) and (3a) shows that in some instances, at least, the particular choice of verb influences performance. We must incorporate linguistic notions to the account of the observed pattern of selectivity. I have made one such proposal (Grodzinsky, 1986), which I will review briefly. But first, some syntactic background is necessary.

Consider the case of passive. One target for the theory of syntax is the contrast in form between sentences like (1a) and (2a), in spite of their similar meanings. This observation, in fact, is a central issue and a source of debate in contemporary linguistics, a debate to which we will return later. For now, I will assume one theoretical approach to passive, the one taken by government and binding theory (Chomsky, 1981 and subsequent literature). According to this theory the grammar consists of several levels of representation with rules of mapping between them; for example, transformational rules. Each level is subject to various conditions of well-formedness. A string is well-formed just in case it does not violate any such condition at any level.

Back to actives and passives. Active sentences are represented in GB theory by tree structures such as in (4):

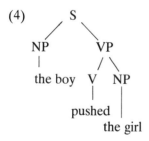

(4)

Grammatical functions (subject, object) and ultimately thematic roles (agent, patient, goal) are read off this representation, which is among the reasons for the structural asymmetry between the first and second NP in the string. The representation of actives like this is the same at all levels. This, however, is not the case for passives. In this construction – represented in (5), the object of the active counterpart (*the girl* in this case) has been moved transformationally into the subject–preverbal position, while leaving an abstract symbol — *trace* in its original position.

(5)

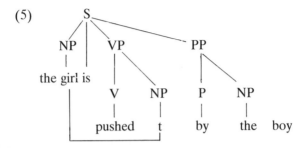

The transformation mapped the deep (D) structure representation onto surface (S) structure. The trace is linked to the new position that the moved NP now occupies. The subject of the active, namely *the boy*, does not replace the object, but is rather attached, as a part of the *by* phrase, to the root S node.

So, a representation of a passive sentence would be this familiar tree structure, with a special link between the subject and the object position. It is this link that is crucial to thematic role assignment to the NPs by the predicate. The verb *push* always assigns its roles in the same fashion, regardless of whether the sentence is in active or in passive. We now focus on the assignment of the theme role. In the former case it is assigned directly to the object, whereas in the passive it is assigned to the trace and transmitted to the subject via the link connecting these two NPs. It is precisely this fact that we can exploit for the formal account of agrammatic comprehension.

Suppose that the only impairment to representations created by the agrammatic comprehension device is that traces are deleted, and that subsequently, thematic roles assigned to it cannot pass to the subject. Suppose, further, that an NP that does not have a grammatically assigned thematic role is assigned one by a heuristic.

(6)

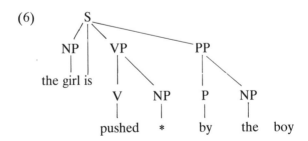

In this case it would be an Agent-first strategy, as proposed by Bever (1970). What would be the outcome for the comprehension of passives? The subject NP in (6) is assigned agenthood by the heuristic; the oblique object, however, is assigned agenthood by the grammar. We now have two agents, and the patient is forced to guess, thereby performing at chance. This problem does not arise in actives, since there are no traces in their representations.

We have thus accounted for the active–passive performance contrast in the comprehension of agrammatic aphasics. Their results on other constructions are derived similarly. Importantly, the chance performance on the relative clauses in (2c–d), in which a Wh-movement transformation applies, is accounted for. This fact will be central to my argument later on. The reader is referred to Grodzinsky (1986) for a full, detailed account. Important to note at this point, however, is that the account proposed really serves as a discovery procedure. It was formulated precisely on the basis of some data, and then motivated further experimentation. Indeed, many of the results listed in (1)–(3) were found after its formulation, which helped us zero in on just the relevant constructions, rather than fish for findings in an undirected way.

It must be stressed that this informally presented account is by no means a comprehensive account of agrammatism as a syndrome. Rather it is a precise, theoretically driven descriptive generalisation of the syntactic deficit. Still, there is one lesson to be learned already at this stage: descriptions of grammatically selective language deficits, such as the one we have in front of us, must incorporate linguistic notions if they are ever to be precise. This immediately excludes theories that focus just on activities — reading, writing, listening and so on, or accounts that assume a complex array of processing devices without making explicit ties to grammatical representations and their properties. That is, if there are performance distinctions in aphasia that correlate with grammatical distinctions, then any account failing to accommodate these is false. But all this is just half of the story. In fact the less exciting one to me, personally. The other half concerns neuropsychological contributions to linguistics and here, I think, is where the action is.

There has been, in the past decade or so, a lot of brouhaha in cognitive science in relation to the so-called psychological reality of theories of grammatical representation. There have been, generally, three such considerations: first, it has been reasoned that if a theory of grammar is a theory of knowledge people have about their language, then, given that this knowledge is not completely innate, the language-specific portion of the grammar has to be learnable by humans (see Wexler and Culicover, 1980). This regards the issue raised above by the question 'how does knowledge of language arise in the individual?'. A realistic theory, then, has to meet the learnability constraint. Second, if a grammar is taken to be the basis for our analysis of incoming sentences, then there must exist an algorithm that can parse sentences in the manner of the grammar as fast as we do, so as to answer the question about use. This imposes on grammars the parsability constraint (see Gazdar, 1981). Third, it has been argued that grammatical theory must account for various and sundry findings from real-time processing (see Fodor, Bever and Garrett, 1974; Bresnan, 1978). I would like to argue for a fourth constraint, one that is motivated by observations on selective impairments to linguistic ability after brain damage (see Grodzinsky, 1985b). Specifically, if the theory of grammar is taken to be about a mentally represented entity, then this theory must reflect the manner by which this mental faculty breaks down. In other words, a grammatical theory must be able to predict the grammatical patterns of selectivity observed in aphasia. If it can account for these in a natural fashion, it will be said to meet the breakdown compatibility constraint. If *ad hoc* devices are necessary for the account, we can reject the theory on the grounds that it is not biologically feasible. Many such constraints may be discovered, of course. I will give one example.

In my discussion of passive, I mentioned a debate among grammarians concerning the correct analysis of this construction. There are, generally, two schools of thought regarding this issue: the first, represented by lexical functional grammar (Bresnan, 1982) and generalized phrase structure grammar (Gazdar, Klein, Pullum and Sag, 1985), sees all passives as derived by a lexical — as opposed to transformational — rule. On this view the derivation of all passives is by a mechanism distinct from that deriving questions, relative clauses and other so-called 'unbounded dependencies'. The other approach, that of government binding, gives passive a 'mixed' analysis: some are derived transformationally in the manner described above, and some are lexical. Unbounded dependencies are derived by a transformation, which means that they are similar to the transformationally derived pasives in the sense that their S-structure representations all contain traces. In the example in (7), LFG and GPSG would derive (7a–b) by a lexical rule, and (7c) by some other transformation-like mechanism, whereas GB, with the mixed analysis of passive, would derive (7a) by a lexical rule, and (7b–c) by a transformation.

			GB	LFG–GPSG
(7)	(a)	John was interested in Mary	lexical	lexical
	(b)	John was killed by Mary	syntactic	lexical
	(c)	The man who Mary pushed was tall	syntactic	syntactic

Each of the two theory types divides the constructions in (7) into two natural classes, yet in a different way. GB cannot state a generalisation over (7a–b), as distinct from (7c). LFG and GPSG, on the other hand, cannot distinguish (7a) from (7b–c). This difference may have consequences for agrammatism. We know already that sentences such as (7b–c) are problematic for agrammatic patients. If the patients were to have problems on examples like (7a), then both theories could handle this finding. Yet if (7a) were found to be comprehended well by the patients, this would mean that the natural class defined by GB theory, and only this theory, can account for the pattern of selectivity. Were this to be the case, then the other two theories could be rejected on the grounds that they fail to meet this constraint.

These considerations guided the experimental search for the breakdown compatibility constraint. With Amy Pierce (Grodzinsky and Pierce, forthcoming), I have been testing patients' comprehension of reversible sentences with structures similar to those in (7). So far, the data suggest that the pattern predicted by GB is indeed the one agrammatic patients follow. This theory is thus the only breakdown-compatible one.

We can thus see how a descriptive generalization over an observed pattern of impairment (stated in structural terms) can be used to motivate a constraint on linguistic theories. Hopefully this particular case is not the only one that can be formulated via the use of neuropsychological data. Our task in the future is to discover performance patterns, and use them for the formulation of other neurologically based constraints on theories of language structure.

I have thus demonstrated how data from agrammatism are treated from a linguistic point of view, and how they can inform linguistic theories. Having made my case I should now consider briefly some potential objections.

It might be argued that the description of agrammatism is based on just a subset of the available data. If this is the case, the argument runs, then we might be dealing with a set of arbitrarily selected facts, which cannot be used to motivate a theoretical constraint. From a different angle it might be argued that the patients whose behaviours are the basis for the argument are selected arbitrarily, or at least not on theoretical grounds. A theoretical account of such a group is thus worthless, on this view. This argument is invalid, however. The only way to select domains is by a theory. In constructing a theory we always use our intuitions as for what is relevant and what isn't, and then propose an account. The relative uniformity of their performance on the task in question, as attested by the experiments I reviewed above, gives us good reasons to believe that agrammatic patients, who might be different from one another in some respects, are similar in their comprehension abilities. Also, it is quite clear that the syntactic abilities of these patients, as evidenced by their comprehension patterns, may be relevant to the theory of syntax and that, by contrast, the fact that many of them are hemiplegic is beside the point. Theories, after all, are nothing more than a formal explication of our intuitions, which we use in science all the time. Thus arguments like this simply miss the point.

So, I believe that I have demonstrated the bidirectional nature of the relation between linguistic theory and neuropsychological phenomena. On the one hand, theories are used as descriptive frameworks of language deficits; on the other, breakdown patterns observed after brain damage are used to motivate constraints on theories of grammatical representation. I have given one example. Many others are probably waiting out there to be discovered.

ACKNOWLEDGEMENT

The preparation of this manuscript was supported by NIH grants NS 06209, 11408 and 21806, and by the Charles Smith Foundation at the Israel Institute for Psychobiology. A version of this paper was read at a

symposium on language deficits and theories of grammatical representation and processing, at the Academy of Aphasia, Nashville, Tenn.,
1986. Address all correspondence to Yosef Grodzinsky, Department of
Linguistics, Tel Aviv University, Ramat Aviv, Tel Aviv 69978, Israel.

REFERENCES

Bever, T.G. (1970) The cognitive basis of linguistic structures. In J.R.
    Hayes (eds), *Cognition and the development of language*, Wiley,
    New York
Bresnan, J. (1978) A realistic transformational grammar. In J. Bresnan,
    M. Halle and G.A. Miller (eds), *Linguistic theory and psychological
    reality*, MIT Press, Cambridge, Mass.
Bresnan, J. (1982) The passive in lexical theory. In J. Bresnan (ed.),
    The mental representation of grammatical relations, MIT Press,
    Cambridge, Mass.
Caplan, D. and Futter, C. (1986) Assignment of thematic roles by an
    agrammatic aphasic patient. *Brain and Language, 27*, 117–35
Caramazza, A and Zurif, E.B. (1976) Dissociation of algorithmic and
    heuristic processes in language comprehension: evidence from
    aphasia. *Brain and Language, 3*, 572–82
Chomsky, N. (1981), *Lectures on government and binding*, Foris,
    Dordrecht
Chomsky, N. (1986) *Knowledge of language*, Praeger, New York
Chomsky, N. and Miller, G.A. (1963) An introduction to the formal
    analysis of language. In R.D. Luce, R.R. Bush and E. Galanter
    (eds), *Readings in mathematical pyschology*, vol. II, Wiley, New
    York
Fodor, J.A., Bever, T.G. and Garret, M.F. (1974) *The psychology of
    language*, McGraw-Hill, New York
Gazdar, G. (1981) Unbounded dependencies and coordinate structure.
    Linguistic Inquiry, 12, 155–84
Gazdar, G., Klein, E., Pullum, G. and Sag, I. (1985) *Generalized
    phrase structure grammar*, Cambridge University Press, Cambridge
Geschwind, N. (1979) Specializations of the human brain. *Scientific
    American*, September
Goodglass, H. and Kaplan, E. (1972) *The assessment of aphasia and
    related disorders*, Lea & Febiger, Philadelphia
Grodzinsky, Y. (1985a) Neurological constraints on models of language
    use. MIT Center for Cognitive Science, Occasional Paper 30,
    Cambridge, Mass.
Grodzinsky, Y. (1985b) On the interaction between linguistics and
    neuropsychology. Review of Noam Chomsky on the generative
    enterprise. *Brain and Language, 26*, 186–96
Grodzinsky, Y. (1986) Language deficits and the theory of syntax.
    Brain and Language, 27, 135–59
Grodzinsky, Y., Finkelstein, D., Nicol, J. and Zurif, E.B. (1985)
    Perceptual strategies and syntactic parsing. Manuscript, MIT and

Aphasia Research Center, Boston

Grodzinsky, Y. and Pierce, A. (forthcoming) Lexical and syntactic passive in agrammatism

Jackendoff, R. (1972) *Semantic interpretation in generative grammar*, MIT Press, Cambridge, Mass

Pick, A. (1913) *Die Agrammatischen Sprachstörungen*, Springer, Berlin

Schwartz, M., Saffran, E. and Marin, O. (1980) The word-order problem in agrammatism: I. Comprehension. *Brain and Language, 10*, 249–62

Wexler, K. and Culicover, P. (1980) *Formal principles of language acquisition*, MIT Press, Cambridge, Mass.

Zurif, E.B. and Caramazza, A. (1976) Psycholinguistic structures in aphasia: studies in syntax and semantics. In H. Whitaker and H.A. Whitaker (eds), *Studies in neurolinguistics*, vol. II, Academic Press, New York

3

Processing Language Breakdown

Shula Chiat and Eirian V. Jones

Stephen, a child with disordered phonological output, is both able and yet unable to produce the phoneme /k/; while he can produce a velar in the words 'record' (noun) and 'back out', he cannot do so in the words 'record' (verb), 'become' and 'be caught'. G.E., an aphasic patient, can say the plural marker 's' in the noun 'cuts', but is not able even to repeat the third person singular 's' in the verb 'cuts'. Such paradoxes are typical of language disorders.

To the psycholinguist the observed behaviours are only superficially paradoxical; the theoretical challenge is to resolve the apparent paradox. This means identifying what distinguishes the cases where the patient can do something from those where he can't. Linguistics provides us with the concepts for describing these distinctions, and psycholinguistics with the theory and methods for identifying them. On the basis of psycholinguistic analysis of pathological language behaviour, inferences can be made about the intact and impaired processing of the patient, and these in turn have implications for the structure of normal language processing.

In this chapter we consider the assumptions, methods and implications of psycholinguistic research into language pathology. The above cases, and others, are developed further in a critical discussion of the current information-processing approach to language pathology, pointing towards new theoretical and methodological challenges for this approach.

LANGUAGE PATHOLOGY AND NORMAL LANGUAGE
PROCESSING; ASSUMPTIONS, QUESTIONS AND METHODS

The advent of cognitive neuropsychology and psycholinguistics has generated a new interest in language disorder. The identification of syndromes permitting clinical diagnosis is no longer the primary objective of investigation. Instead, the objective is a theory of language processing which accounts for both normal and pathological language behaviours. This shift of interest has been most explicit, and has had most effects, in the study of adult dyslexia and aphasia; it is these disorders which have stimulated neuropsychological and psycholinguistic research. However, such research is equally relevant to developmental disorders of language processing. We start off by exploring the assumptions behind this research, the methodology it employs and the theoretical models which arise from it.

The starting point for such research is the assumption that normal language processing is modular, involving a system of distinct components or modules, each of which performs particular computations over a particular type of code (e.g. Morton and Patterson, 1980; Caramazza and Berndt, 1985; Coltheart, 1985; Howard and Patterson, in press). These modules receive the visual or auditory stimuli of language, and map this onto semantic representations, or conversely, map semantic representations into visual or auditory output. A cognitive process such as reading a word is modelled in terms of the types of information about the word, or codes, which are available at different stages between the input of the visual stimulus and the retrieval of the word's semantics. It is further assumed that the system of processing components engaged in cognitive processes is universal (Caramazza, 1986). That is, the structure of cognitive processes does not vary from individual to individual. Language disorder is then construed as a breakdown in this universal system which affects certain components and spares others. The goal of current neuropsychological or psycholinguistic accounts of language behaviour is to specify the components involved in language input and output processing, the nature of the representations they process, and the nature of breakdown in their functioning.

An information-processing theory therefore seeks to explain normal and pathological language behaviour, and must be compatible with data from both. The relevance of pathological data is that they provide evidence for the discreteness of different aspects of processing. If one behaviour is intact, while another is impaired, it may be assumed that the processes underlying those behaviours are distinct. A classic example is the case of a patient who can read words but not non-words, or one who can read regular words and non-words, but not irregular words, implying different processing routes in the reading of these different types of words. The first case points to a 'visual route' which permits reading of familiar words, and a 'phonological route' which permits reading of unfamiliar words and which is impaired in this patient. In the second case the inability to read irregular words suggests that the patient has no access to the visual route which is required to read irregular words, and is relying on the phonological route to read regular words.

These assumptions and goals in the study of language pathology favour a single-case methodology. Dissociations between intact and impaired processes can only be identified within a single system; what matters is that there is a discrepancy for a single patient. On the assumption of a universal processing system it is enough to show that one system exists where a dissociation between functions occurs to infer the discreteness of those functions within the universal processing system. If even one patient can read words but not non-words, the system must allow distinct processing for these. Where a number of patients exhibit the same dissociation, the evidence for discrete functions is reinforced. But such reinforcement is provided by a series of single case studies rather than by traditional group studies. Group studies seek statistically valid generalisations about groups of patients, and these cannot throw light on possible dissociations and hence on discrete components of language processing.

The approach we have briefly outlined has generated models of information-processing. These are most developed for single word reading, (e.g. Coltheart, Patterson and Marshall, 1980). However, the information-processing approach is extending to the processing of spoken language, and underlies much current research into symptoms such as agrammatic output (e.g. Saffran, 1982), word deafness (e.g. Caramazza, Berndt and Basili, 1983), or word-finding problems (e.g. Morton, 1985). In these cases, where the production and comprehension of words and sentences are at stake, the models are less explicit than those which characterise single word reading. Nevertheless, they reflect the same assumptions and methods, seeking to describe the linguistic representations which are impaired (phonological, semantic or syntactic) and/or the stage of processing which is impaired (storage or accessing in input or output); relating these to models of normal processing (e.g. Garrett's model of production (1982)); and advancing them as evidence for such models (e.g. Butterworth, 1980, 1983).

In contrast to adult language pathology, child language pathology has remained relatively untouched by developments in neuropsychology and psycholinguistics. Pathologies such as developmental phonological delay or disorder, or developmental aphasia, have rarely been considered as disruptions in the language processing system which may be informed by and contribute to theories of language processing. Instead, assessment and research on these disorders has been largely confined to linguistic description of deviant phonology, syntax or semantics (Bloom and Lahey, 1978; Grunwell, 1981; Ingram, 1981; Crystal, 1982), or has sought to identify diagnostic criteria (Wyke, 1978; Bishop and Rosenbloom, in press). There has been little attempt at single-case studies which investigate constraints in the process of mapping between semantics, syntax and phonological input/output.

LIMITATIONS OF CURRENT MODELS

The thrust of this chapter is not to question the general theoretical objectives of the information-processing approach, with its identification of normal and pathological language processing as a theoretical domain, and its single-case methodology. On the contrary, we assume this approach and advocate its extension to the study of childhood pathologies. Our contribution starts from this approach but takes issue with some of the further assumptions, methods and theoretical constructs which have emerged within it.

The models developed within the information-processing approach depend crucially on the theoretical concepts and the methods available to identify intact and impaired processing, and are only as sophisticated as these. We suggest that current conceptual and methodological machinery is simplistic in certain respects, generating correspondingly simplistic theoretical models. Data emerging within the current framework are not compatible with these simplistic models, and begin to point beyond this framework.

Apart from assuming a universal processing system, information-processing approaches to language pathology make a further assumption: in Caramazza's terms (1986), that the processing of a brain-damaged patient is the same as that of a normal subject apart from 'local' modification; or for Coltheart (1985), that a certain subset of components is damaged within a multicomponent information-processing system. It is this assumption which allows extrapolation from dissociations in the pathological system to discrete functions in the normal system. We would question this assumption and its justification, on theoretical and empirical grounds. We would not assume that the pathological system is totally unrelated or arbitrarily related to the normal system, i.e. that brain damage results in a qualitatively new system for processing language. However, the relation between the two may well be less direct than is assumed. It seems likely that damage to one part of a system may have knock-on effects, since the system must adjust to the damage. We are not, here, referring to conscious adaptations on the part of the patient, but to automatic adjustments of a system to exploit connections between intact functions in novel ways. This would produce behaviours which do not directly reflect the normal interconnections of the processing system. In this case, inferences from dissociations in the pathological behaviour to discrete functions in the normal system are not justified. This may be illustrated by the hypothetical case of patients whose access to the phonological representation for certain types of words is impaired. The patient's system may respond to this impairment in two different ways: by omitting those words, or by filling in the unknowns with arbitrary phonology (producing 'jargon'). The patient's output then compounds the underlying problem with the adjustment of the system to that problem. Observation of the patient's output allows a variety of interpretations, yielding a variety of inferences about the nature of the processing system and its breakdown. We may interpret the jargon as evidence of damage to some phonological component, and the omissions as evidence of damage to some syntactic component. But as we have already seen, both are equally interpretable in terms of a single site of damage together with different adjustments of the system. The relation between pathological behaviour and normal processing may, then, be

35

somewhat less direct than is generally assumed. We are not denying this relation altogether, however. We are simply pointing out a certain complexity which means that we require subtle concepts and methods to break into the ambiguity of pathological behaviour and make inferences about the nature of the damaged and normal systems.

Current concepts and methods match this oversimplifying assumption. Typically, investigations into language processing seek to identify linguistically discrete impairments. Typically, they do so by presenting the patient with linguistically controlled input stimuli within some task where the accuracy or speed of the patient's response may reflect the differences controlled for in the input. In spoken language tasks, patients are frequently required to judge linguistic stimuli as same/different or correct/incorrect, to match them to pictures, to complete them, to correct them, and so on, in order to determine whether some aspect of language is preserved at a particular stage of processing. The stimuli are controlled for that aspect of language, which may be syntactic, semantic or phonological. For example, a patient may be required to judge sentences which are correct, semantically anomalous, or syntactically ill-formed, in order to assess her input syntax and semantics. The results from such tasks yield conclusions about the aspects of language which are impaired and the stage of input–output at which they are impaired, and hence point to components and subcomponents of the processing system. The outcome of these investigations is a model or fragment of a model of language processing which consists of boxes (components of language processing) and arrows (the interconnections between these components). We suggest that these 'boxes and arrows' models reflect the starting assumptions we have outlined, and are in some respects an artefact of them. If one assumes discretely affected functions, and designs tasks to distinguish functions, these will indicate discrete functions in the performance of the tasks; but they may obscure interconnections between functions within the patient's spontaneous language processing system.

This possibility follows from the methodological and theoretical assumptions discussed above. First, the tasks designed to elicit measurable responses from the patient are typically off-line tasks, i.e. they require conscious reflection on a word or sentence, in order to make a judgement about it or match it to another stimulus. They therefore probe metalinguistic processes, which follow automatic language comprehension or production, rather than tapping the automatic processes of language comprehension and production as these take place. This is not to undermine the evidence from such tasks, which often reveal systematic differences between patients' responses and normal responses, and point up further questions about the nature of the deficit. The question is what they are evidence of. It cannot be assumed that variables shown to be significant in an off-line task are also critical in on-line processing. The point has recently been well made by Tyler (forthcoming). She has developed a technique for tapping certain on-line processes, and provides evidence that a patient may show different patterns of response to a particular variable in off-line and on-line tasks. It may be, then, that discrete components of processing are a function of metalinguistic rather than linguistic processing.

Under the impetus to identify discrete representations in processing, these off-line tasks explore the role of particular aspects of language independently of one another. Frequently the question asked of a patient's system is: which level of language (phonology, syntax or semantics), and what type of structure within these levels, is implicated by the patient's behaviour? If it is possible to provide a linguistic description of intact and impaired structures which distinguishes systematically between these, the linguistic characterisation of the impairment is interpreted as a psycholinguistic representation which has been lost or can no longer be retrieved. The linguistic description is therefore elevated to a psycholinguistic explanation. The study of agrammatism provides a good example: there has been much debate as to whether the disorder is phonological, syntactic or semantic, with researchers attempting to show that the errors and omissions involved are best described at one or another of these levels.

We do not question the importance of linguistic description in psycholinguistic research. It is only through linguistic description that we can begin to specify questions about psycholinguistic processing. Without linguistic concepts we have no conceptual tools for describing the phenomena observed in language behaviour: we could not begin to distinguish what a patient can and cannot do. Furthermore, the more sophisticated the linguistic concepts at our disposal, the more chance we have of picking out significant generalisations about a patient's language input and output. However, we would question the status of linguistic description in psycholinguistic research. Linguistic concepts are part of a theory about language systems in the abstract, and not about real-time language processing. It is not necessarily the case that distinctions which are well motivated on linguistic grounds are critical factors in language processing (cf. Black and Chiat, 1981, for further discussion about the independence of linguistic argumentation, and the role of linguistics in psycholinguistic theory). A similar point is made by Caramazza and Berndt, who identify the concern of psycholinguistic theory as the computations in real-time processes which 'will bear some relationship to the formal, linguistic description of a language (the grammar)', but 'are not isomorphic with such descriptions' (Caramazza and Berndt, 1985, p. 28).

Again, the identification of discretely affected represent-ations may be an artefact of the question asked. Task materials are designed in such a way as to differentiate linguistic factors, so that crucial interactions between them may fail to be revealed.

It may well be, then, that current theorisation about the structures of the language processing system and their selective impairment follow from the assumption that components of language processing function independently, break down independently and may be identified on the basis of indepen-dent behaviour in off-line tasks. If we set out from the assump-tion that language processing involves integrated and mutually dependent processes, where breakdown in a particular aspect may trigger adjustments within the system, and we explore the interactions within the system, we may come up with inform-ation-processing models which are rather different from current 'boxes and arrows'.

Such is the theoretical rationale for seeking new develop-ments in language pathology. Empirical evidence reinforces this. While 'boxes and arrows' models are consistent with certain observed behaviours, most notably in the case of single-word reading in normal and dyslexic subjects, other behaviours defy interpretation in terms of such models. Investigation into word and sentence processing in spoken language rarely reveals the neat patterns of dissociation which occur in reading disor-ders. Patients frequently show variability rather than an all-or-nothing response to a particular linguistic factor. For example, agrammatic patients tend to miss out function words, but it is not predictable whether a particular word or function words in general will be omitted. Such inconsistency is not easily reconciled with a model in which a box or arrow is either intact or impaired. If we are to throw light on the system which gives rise to such inconsistency, we need to consider what variables may affect the availability of a word or structure in on-line processing, to determine whether there are underlying patterns with implications for the nature of language processing. This may mean looking at the interaction of linguistic variables, rather than seeking to dissociate them.

In line with this suggestion, evidence is beginning to emerge in studies of normal language development which points to interdependence between 'information' which would be processed in separate 'boxes' according to current information-processing models. A recent study by Caramata and Leonard (1985), for example, indicates that the articulation of a word is not independent of its syntax: children's ability to articulate a sound within a word was observed to vary according to the syntactic category of the word. Similar observations about an adult with acquired language disorder will be discussed below. These suggest that syntactic role and the organisation of articulation may interact in ways which are difficult to explain within a 'boxes and arrows' model. Such a model could conceivably include direct connections between, for example, a syntactic component and articulation. However, it could not account for the specificity of the influence, i.e. that a category *within* the syntactic component affects articulation.

We suggest that advances can only be made if we devise techniques for tapping on-line processing, and use these to investigate the ways in which different aspects of language interact in language processing. Methodologically, this means relying less on tasks such as judgement and picture matching, and more on tasks which elicit responses which are contingent upon automatic processing but require no reflection on it. Theoretically, it means predicting which aspects of language processing may interact, investigating these, and developing models which account for observed interactions.

SOME EVIDENCE OF INTERACTIONS BETWEEN
LANGUAGE COMPONENTS

Current models of language processing assume the discreteness of semantics and phonology: language input and output involve the mapping from one component to another, and the theoretical goal is to specify the components and their internal structure. We have suggested that different types of information, such as phonological and semantic information, are not necessarily discrete components in on-line input and output processing. In this section we consider some evidence from language-disordered patients which indicates the role of semantic factors in phonological output. Such evidence is difficult to explain in terms of a model with discrete, ordered components, where one component receives the output from another component, but does not have access to the internal structure of that component.

Delayed or deviant phonology in children is generally considered as a problem in the child's phonological system, rather than in the process of phonological output. Even though most children diagnosed as having these problems show intact perception of phonological distinctions which are neutralised in their output, the neutralisation of phonemic contrast is attributed to their internal phonological system. For the psycholinguist, the interesting question is where the child is and is not able to make a contrast, and what the implications are for the organisation of phonological storage and output. A study of a child's velar fronting (Chiat, 1983) indicated that the child's velars were fronted depending on their position relative to stress and word boundaries: fronting occurred in all word-initial velars, e.g. *case, can, collect,* and in pre-stressed word-medial velars, e.g. *forget, again*; in other positions, i.e. in word-final and post-stressed word-medial positions, velars were correct. The effect of word boundaries gives rise to minimal pairs such as *back out* vs. *because, bacon* vs. *they can* (with *can* reduced to [kən]), where the child can realise the velar in the first but not in the second member of these pairs. Clearly, he can articulate the target velar in the phonological contexts where he fronts them, since he does articulate the velar in contexts which are phonologically identical in relevant respects. His differentiation of these contexts indicates that velar fronting, which affects articulation, operates in the phonological context of word units rather than phonological strings of words. This suggests that words, rather than phonological strings which are semantically and syntactically unsegmented, are the units for at least some aspects of articulatory organisation. The conclusions that can be drawn from these data remain tentative, and await elaboration on the basis of further investigation into the factors which condition children's phonological deviations. However, they do point to the possibility that in on-line processing there may be a direct mapping from word semantics/syntax to articulatory programming, rather than a mapping from a syntactically organised sequence of words to a phonological representation to articulatory programming.

Further evidence for this may also come from adult patients with acquired language disorders. G.E., a non-fluent aphasic patient, can generate and articulate with ease the plural marker 's', for example in the noun 'cuts'. However, he is totally unable to articulate, even in repetition tasks, the equivalent form when marking the third person singular, for example in the verb 'cuts'. It may not be immediately obvious that this is an articulatory problem. Before judging it as such there are a number of other explanations that need to be considered. Omission of the verb inflection could reflect a syntactic error. However, G.E. is able to make grammaticality judgements, uses the form correctly in written output, and indicates monitoring of this error by saying that the letter 's' is missing. The problem could also arise because of difficulty in accessing the phonological information. Omission of a verb inflection is in line with Kean's theory (1979, 1980) that agrammatic output can be accounted for by the fact that such items are clitics. If this were the case, the plural marker 's' should also be a problem, which it clearly is not. Difficulty in accessing segmental information could also account for the omission. This is particularly the case as G.E., although showing no phonological errors, either segmental or suprasegmental, in input, makes a number of phonemic errors in output. However, if this were the explanation, he should still be able to repeat the verb. Although he can repeat the phoneme /s/ and the cluster /ts/ in isolation, he repeats the phrase 'he cuts' as 'he cut' but 'many cuts' is repeated correctly. Despite repeated efforts, G.E. cannot articulate the phoneme /s/ as part of the verb 'cuts'. It appears that, for this patient, articulation of inflectional markers is dependent on the syntactic representation they encode.

The role of pragmatic bias in allowing patients to by-pass syntactic processing is well recognised, for example where pragmatic knowledge is sufficient to identify the role of noun arguments (Caramazza and Zurif, 1976). However, such a view of the role of pragmatics may be too simplistic. An experiment by Jones (1984) suggests that even where pragmatic factors are not sufficient to by-pass syntactic processing, they may still facilitate it. The first task in the experiment was designed to assess aphasic patients' ability to process the grammatical relations marked by a directional motion verb such as 'chase' when placed in a simple active reversible sentence such as 'The policeman chases the fireman'. Patients were asked to select one of three pictures in which the target sentence was depicted, together with its reverse role ('The fireman chases the policeman'), and a distractor picture where the noun arguments of the target were depicted carrying out a different activity (e.g. 'The policeman photographs the fireman'). When such complex verbs were used, Wernicke's patients found the processing load of this task so great that they sometimes picked the distractor picture, which suggests that they had not accessed any information about the correct verb. However, in a second task where the verb 'chase' was placed in a pragmatically biased sentence, e.g. 'The policeman chases the thief', they made neither distractor nor reversal errors. Initially it may appear unsurprising that they could perform correctly in this task. They could have by-passed any linguistic processing by choosing the most likely picture. However, this could not have been the case since the distractor picture in this task depicted an equally plausible relationship between the arguments, e.g.

The policeman chases the thief: Target.
The thief chases the policeman: Reverse.
The policeman handcuffs the thief: Distractor.

If they had been responding on the basis of the 'most likely' alone, there would have been an equal chance of them selecting the distractor. Their correct selection of the target indicates that choosing between two pragmatically plausible pictures in this task was easier than choosing between unrelated pictures in the first task, where pragmatic bias was eliminated. It would appear that the pragmatic bias in the second task enhanced linguistic processing, since verb information previously inaccessible to the patients was now available. It seems, then, that the availability of semantic information about a verb is not independent of other knowledge sources. The pragmatic bias in this task did not in any way identify the semantics of the verb, yet its presence still affected the availability of that semantic information.

FUTURE DIRECTIONS

We have argued that current information-processing models are simplistic in certain respects. However, we recognise that without the seminal work undertaken to formulate such models, including linguistic description of spontaneous behaviour and responses in off-line processing tasks, we would not be in a position to identify the questions we are now raising. Furthermore, while modular approaches to language breakdown assume and aim to specify discrete components within the language-processing system, they do not deny the interaction between modules (e.g. Berndt and Caramazza, 1981; Howard and Patterson, in press). The position is made particularly clear by Caramazza and Berndt (1985):

> The characterization of the modules that make up the language processing system as independent of one another should not be translated into a claim about the nature of the relationship among these modules in on-line language processing. The independence of the modules is determined strictly on the basis of the assumptions one makes about the computations and codes that are presumed to characterize a particular process ... the claim that processes are interactive in on-line processing is not incompatible with the notion that the modules are independent (Caramazza and Berndt, 1985, pp. 28-9).

The interaction between modules may even obscure the discrete role each plays in normal and pathological language behaviours (Howard and Patterson, in press). Given this possibility, it could be argued that the interactions we have discussed above reflect interactions between language processing components, and do not undermine the discreteness of these components. In other words we have simply shifted the focus from 'boxes' to 'arrows', from modules to the interaction between modules. The arrows still presuppose the boxes: the interactions are premised upon discrete modules which interact.

Contrary to this interpretation, we would argue that the assumptions and evidence we have advanced represent a substantially different conception of language processing and language breakdown within an information-processing approach. They do not reduce to a mere change of emphasis. Current research sets out to find dissociated functions and postulate discrete components, and the interaction between these components in on-line processing is secondary to the discreteness of their computations and codes. In contrast, we have identified on-line processing as the crucial object of psycholinguistic investigation; we have argued that on-line processing rarely reveals clear-cut dissociations, showing variability in performance of a particular process which can only be explained in terms of the interaction between different types of information or codes. Can the modular approach account for phenomena of the type we have discussed?

One possibility would be to explain the effects of one component on another in terms of further psychological mechanisms, such as a working memory which may itself be modular. Caramazza and Berndt (1985), for example, postulate modular working memories, such that a memory limitation which disrupts processing within one module might limit the input to a different module. However, attributing interactions between modules to the effects of modular working memories would imply a quantitative limitation on the output of one module and hence the input to another. It is difficult to see how such a quantitative limitation could account for the interactions we have described, where there is a qualitative interaction between different types of code. An alternative possibility would be to allow a module to contain different types of information, such as pragmatic and syntactic information, or to allow connections (arrows) between specific information within separate modules. In our view these modifications conflict with the fundamental assumption of discrete information-processing modules, each performing distinct computations over distinct codes. Once one 'box' has access to the internal structure of another, or computes more than one code, there is no longer a clear distinction between 'boxes' containing codes and 'arrows' linking these. Language behaviour is no longer the product of computations over discrete representations, carried out serially or in parallel; instead, it is the product of dialectically related representations, where a computation over one code is affected by a computation over a different code.

We suggest that the difference between these conceptions is reflected in the questions they raise about child and adult language disorders, the methods used to address these questions and the implications for clinical intervention.

The area of agrammatism provides a good example of the different questions which may follow from the general perspective we have advocated. As we pointed out above, research into agrammatism has been much concerned with the linguistic description of agrammatic errors and omissions: whether these reflect a phonological, syntactic or semantic deficit (Kean, 1979, 1980; Saffran, 1982; Schwartz, Linebarger and Saffran, 1985). Psycholinguistic analyses of the disorder consider the storage and retrieval processes of items or structures at the relevant level. As yet, no description has been clearly shown to be more adequate than another, and there is still much debate about the most appropriate level of description. This may simply be because our linguistic descriptions are not sophisticated enough, or our psycholinguistic evidence detailed enough, to resolve the issue. We suggest that the problem is not only the sophistication of description or data. Any analysis at a particular linguistic level predicts a neat pattern of language breakdown which is not borne out by the data. Agrammatic utterances are not, typically, strings of content words with omission of all function words and grammatical morphemes; agrammatic patients do not consistently omit a particular function word or function words in general, and they often show limited use of content words, especially verbs (Caramazza and Berndt, 1985). This variability could be explained in terms of varying interactions between components in on-line processing, each of which is nevertheless discretely affected. However, if we assume that connections between specific structures at different levels (or in different codes) are primary in on-line processing, and investigate these connections rather than discrete linguistic components, we might gain more insight into the disorder. This concept of mapping between specific structures at different levels has already been considered in relation to word-order problems in agrammatism (Schwartz, Saffran and Marin, 1980; Saffran, Schwartz and Marin, 1980; Jones, 1984). However, its role has not been given the emphasis we are now advocating.

45

Neither has enough consideration been given to mapping between other types of structures. For example, it may be that sentence syntax and sentence phonology are not distinct in on-line processing. That is, the production of a sentence may be a direct mapping from a conceptual intention to a complex rhythmic pattern (see Selkirk, 1984, for an analysis of the relation between sentence syntax and phonology). Agrammatism may then be an impairment in this mapping, which constrains words according to their semantic–phonological role in sentences, and limits the rhythmic structure of the sentence. The interaction between specific semantic and phonological structures may account for the inconsistent pattern of output. In terms of this proposal, which clearly requires elaboration, it is not simply an on-line interaction between modules that is at stake, but the interaction between specific semantic and phonological representations.

In order to investigate the interconnections between specific structures in on-line processing we require techniques which elicit automatic rather than metalinguistic responses. This means devising tasks where the response is contingent on a particular variable, without requiring comparison of stimuli controlled for that variable (as in picture selection), or reflection on such stimuli (as in judgement tasks). We have already mentioned the technique developed by Tyler (1985, forthcoming). This probes on-line processing by asking the patient to monitor a word, and placing that word in different linguistic contexts to determine whether the patient's monitoring is affected by these differences. The critical linguistic variable is not itself under scrutiny in the patient's response, but that response is contingent upon spontaneous processing of the variable. A similar task might require a patient to repeat sentences containing a key word, related to a variable in a prior context, to determine whether that variable affects the patient's repetition. Again, repetition of the variable is not required; repetition is merely used as a possible reflex and measure of the patient's spontaneous processing of the variable in the prior context.

Tasks which probe on-line processing might also be applicable with children. Children's responses to metalinguistic tasks, such as picture selection, often reflect problems in understanding or meeting the task requirements, which may obscure the processing the task is designed to test. On-line tasks involve less extraneous processing and are therefore less vulnerable to interference.

If such methods can be used with children, we are in a position to ask psycholinguistic questions about child language pathologies, which have not previously been considered in relation to models of language processing. For example, rather than debating whether a child is to be diagnosed 'phonetic/ articulatory disorder' or 'phonological disorder', we may ask at what point errors arise in the process of inputting or outputting words, and consider the implications for the processes of speech recognition and production. Similarly, we may go beyond the diagnosis of 'language delay' vs. 'language disorder/developmental aphasia' in children, and investigate where a child's problems arise in the process of mapping between conceptual intentions and their phonological/syntactic realisation. Again, the nature of constraints on the child's mapping will have implications for the nature of the processing system (see Chiat and Hirson (1987) for examples and further discussion).

The development of on-line tasks and the understanding which emerges from them may make psycholinguistic theory more relevant to clinical intervention. Although one might assume that a better understanding of language breakdown would provide a rationale for goals and strategies in intervention, current research has made little impact on therapy. One reason for this is that informal observation of patient performance often denies the results of off-line tasks, leading the clinician to doubt the validity and usefulness of such results. This superficial discrepancy between research findings and clinical observations is not necessarily due to differences in theoretical and methodological rigour. It may reflect the theoretical and methodological limitations which, we have suggested, characterise current research. These limitations mean that such research has few implications for intervention. As we have seen, the goal of research is generally to identify separate modules of the language processing system on the basis of dissociations between specific linguistic variables. The focus is therefore not on on-line processing, which is the concern of the clinician. Furthermore, in seeking dissociations, research identifies what the patient cannot do, but it gives little insight into why, and hence into what remediation is possible. If a patient fails with a particular structure in a task, the implication is that a particular module is impaired. However detailed the specification of the impairment, it does not indicate whether the patient can be retaught the structure; whether the patient is unable to process the structure in the normal way but could access it by novel means; or whether the patient has no means at all of processing the structure. The analysis therefore has no implications for re-teaching, devising novel strategies, or circumvention, which are the alternatives available in clinical intervention. We have suggested a shift in focus from dissociations between variables to interconnections between variables in processing. This means identifying which variables affect each other, as well as which are independent of each other. An understanding of the interactions between variables in a patient's processing system is more likely to reveal which factors facilitate processing, and indicate cues or indirect strategies which the patient may exploit. Conversely, therapy could itself be theoretically informative. Hypotheses about possible interactions could well be forthcoming from observations of patients' reactions to on-line tasks used as therapeutic stimuli.

We opened this chapter with some observations of paradoxes in language pathology. We suggest that the future of the field lies in researching the question raised by such paradoxes. The question is not only what patients can and cannot do, but why patients cannot do what they can do.

REFERENCES

Berndt, R.S. and Caramazza, A. (1981) Syntactic aspects of aphasia. In M.T. Sarno, (ed.), *Acquired aphasia*. Academic Press, New York

Bishop, D.V.M. and Rosenbloom, L. (in press) Classification of child-hood language disorders. In W. Yule, M. Rutter, and M.C.O. Bax. (eds), *Language development and disorders: clinics in developmental medicine*. 101/102, MacKeith Press, London

Black, M. and Chiat, S. (1981) Psycholinguistics without 'psychological reality'. *Linguistics, 19*, 37-61

Bloom, L. and Lahey, M. (1978) *Language development and language disorders*. John Wiley & Sons, New York

Butterworth, B. (ed.) (1980, 1983) *Language production*, vols 1 and 2. Academic Press, London

Caramata, S.M. and Leonard, L.B. (1985) Young children pronounce nouns more accurately than verbs: evidence for a semantic–phonological interaction. *Papers and Reports in Child Language Development, 24*, 38-45

Caramazza, A. (1986) On drawing inferences about the structure of normal cognitive systems from the analysis of patterns of impaired performance: a case for single-patient studies. *Brain and Cognition, 5*, 41-66

Caramazza, A. and Berndt, R.S. (1985) A multicomponent deficit view of agrammatic Broca's aphasia. In M.L. Kean, (ed.). *Agrammatism*, Academic Press, Orlando

Caramazza, A., Berndt, R.S. and Basili, A.G. (1983) The selective impairment of phonological processing: a case study. *Brain and Language, 18*, 128-74

Caramazza, A. and Zurif, E.B. (1976) Dissociation of algorithmic and heuristic processes in language comprehension: evidence from aphasia. *Brain and Language, 3*, 572-82

Chiat, S. (1983) Why *Mikey*'s right and *my key*'s wrong: the significance of stress and word boundaries in a child's output system. *Cognition, 14*, 275-300

Chiat, S. and Hirson, A. (1987) From conceptual intention to utterance: a study of impaired language output in a child with developmental dysphasia. *British Journal of Disorders of Communication, 22*, 37-64

Coltheart, M. (1985) Cognitive neuropsychology and the study of reading. In M.I. Posner, and O.S.M. Marin, (eds), *Attention and performance*, vol. XI, Lawrence Erlbaum, Hillsdale, N.J

Coltheart, M., Patterson, K. and Marshall, J.C. (eds) (1980) *Deep dyslexia*. Routledge & Kegan Paul, London

Crystal, D. (1982) *Profiling linguistic disability*, Edward Arnold, London

Garrett, M.F. (1982) Production of speech: observation from normal and pathological language use. In A. Ellis, (ed), *Normality and pathology in cognitive functions*, Academic Press, London

Grunwell, P. (1981) *The nature of phonological disability in children*, Academic Press, London

Howard, D. and Patterson, K. (in press) Methodological issues in neuropsychological therapy. In X. Seron, and G. Deloche, (eds), *Cognitive approaches in neuropsychological rehabilitation*, Lawrence Erlbaum Associates, Hillsdale, NJ

Ingram, D. (1981) *Procedures for the phonological analysis of children's language*, University Park Press, Baltimore

Jones, E.V. (1984) Word order processing in aphasia: effect of verb semantics. In F.C. Rose, (ed.), *Advances in Neurology*, vol. 42: *Progress in aphasiology*, Raven Press, New York

Kean, M.L. (1979) Agrammatism, a phonological deficit? *Cognition, 7*, 69-83

Kean, M.L. (1980) Grammatical representations and the description of language processes. In D. Caplan, (ed.), *Biological studies of mental processes*, MIT Press, Cambridge, Mass.

Kean, M.L. (1982) Three perspectives for the analysis of aphasic syndromes. In M.A. Arbib, D. Caplan, and J.C. Marshall, (eds), *Neural models of language processes*, Academic Press, New York

Morton, J. (1985) Naming. In S. Newman, and R. Epstein, (eds), *Current perspectives in dysphasia*, Churchill Livingstone, Edinburgh

Morton, J. and Patterson, K. (1980) A new attempt at an interpretation, or, an attempt at a new interpretation. In M. Coltheart, K. Patterson, and J.C. Marshall, (eds), *Deep dyslexia*, Routledge &

Kegan Paul, London

Saffran, E.M. (1982) Neuropsychological approaches to the study of language. *British Journal of Psychology, 73*, 317-37

Saffran, E.M., Schwartz, M.F. and Marin, O.S.M. (1980) The word order problem in agrammatism: II. Production. *Brain and Language, 10*, 263-80

Schwartz, M.F., Linebarger, M.C. and Saffran, E.M. (1985) The status of the syntactic deficit theory of agrammatism. In M.L. Kean (ed.), *Agrammatism*, Academic Press, Orlando

Schwartz, M.F., Saffran, E.M. and Marin, O.S.M. (1980) The word order problem in agrammatism: I. Comprehension. *Brain and Language, 10*, 249-62

Selkirk, E.O. (1984) *Phonology and syntax: the relation between sound and structure*, MIT Press, Cambridge, Mass.

Tyler, L.K. (1985) Real-time comprehension processes in agrammatism: a case study. *Brain and Language, 26*, 259-75

Tyler, L.K. (forthcoming) Locating the comprehension deficit in Wernicke's aphasia

Wyke, M.A. (1978) *Developmental dysphasia*, Academic Press, London

4

Stuttering and Linguistics

Martin Duckworth

INTRODUCTION

Despite the growing pool of knowledge about stuttering, many stutterers in therapy continue to find difficulties in achieving reliable fluency. The intractability of many — if not most — fluency problems leads many therapists to conclude that solving the stuttering problem involves more than reducing the number of stutters to zero. Without the yardstick of fluency, however, it has proved difficult to decide what constitutes successful therapeutic outcome. Opinions differ not only about the definition of successful therapy but about the nature of stuttering and therefore the most appropriate type of intervention. This does not mean to say we have no understanding of the problem for there is much well-documented information about stuttering (e.g. see reviews by Bloodstein, 1981; Van Riper, 1982; Andrews, Craig, Feyer, Hoddinott, Howie and Neilson, 1983). However, this chapter questions whether we have paid sufficient attention to the relationship between speech behaviour and language skills in general, and to the linguistic functions of non-fluency in particular. The functional significance of non-fluency in stuttered and non-stuttered speech may have implications both for the theory and therapy of stuttering.

Psychological interpretations of stuttering — psychodynamic, behavioural, neuropsychological — have had considerable support during the twentieth century (Bloodstein, 1981; Van Riper, 1982; Andrews *et al.*, 1983). Although there are some well-known observations which suggest that moments of stuttering are constrained by factors which have at least as much to do with the structure of language as the psychological processes of people who stutter, there have been relatively few linguistic investigations of stuttering. Indeed, one of the most influential of this century's theories of stuttering — as far as therapeutic practice is concerned — uses linguistic data relating to the typology of fluency disruptions in children and interprets it in terms of the psychology with which its author, Wendell Johnson, was more interested. Johnson (1959) argued that his research (conducted over many years and largely in the form of interviews with parents) showed that the speech of children described as stutterers by their parents did not differ significantly from the speech of children who were not labelled in this way. He hypothesised that the parental labelling of non-fluency as stuttering, which included the reactions of the parents to the non-fluencies, induced the child to attend to the act of speech more closely, thereby inhibiting its automaticity and increasing the likelihood of fluency breakdown. The onset of stuttering was therefore considered to be the result of adult reactions to children's speech and the children's reaction to the parental behaviour. The speech behaviour which prompted the parental diagnosis, as well as the nature of the parental reaction, was not examined empirically. The constraints upon fluency were believed to have more to do with the intrapersonal psychology, particularly of parents, than with the structure and functional use of language: stuttering developed because fluency had a particular salience for these parents and subsequently for the child.

The decline in influence of the Johnsonian theory of stuttering onset has been charted by surveys of American therapists conducted by Cooper and Cooper (1985), who reported that nearly 90 per cent of therapists questioned believed that stuttering was the result of 'multiple coexisting factors' (p. 29). No doubt the evidence cited by writers such as Cooper (1979), Shine (1980) and Ingham (1983), which suggests that calling attention to the stutter, by suggesting to the child strategies for overcoming the break in fluency, may be more of a help than a hindrance to many children with fluency problems has been instrumental in reducing the influence of Johnson's theory. The concurrent development of belief in multiple and coexisting causatory factors may speak as much for the diverse state of the literature on stuttering as for any firm convictions within the therapeutic profession. The period of Cooper and Cooper's (1985) study, i.e. 1973 to 1983, has seen the development of therapeutic programmes which cannot be said to reflect a belief in a multiplicity of factors underlying stuttering (e.g. Ingham and Andrews, 1973; Ryan and Van Kirk, 1978; Shames and Florance, 1980; Shine, 1980). On the other hand, during the same period there have been developed increasingly sophisticated analyses of the neuromotor control of speech and language. This has led to a re-emergence of interest in organic factors in stuttering (Adams, 1985; Kent, 1985; Moore, 1985; Yeudall, 1985) and the therapy programmes mentioned above have been considered *post hoc* as appropriate means of enabling stutterers to overcome these factors (e.g. Boberg, Yeudall, Schopflocher and Bo-Lassen, 1983).

Variability in the occurrence of stuttering appears to be an argument against organicity. Andrews *et al.* (1983) maintained that the empirical evidence actually suggests the relative invariability of stuttering in any one individual, and Yeudall's (1985) neuropsychological theory envisaged that variation could be accounted for as a by-product of the biological cycles of the stutterer. To suggest that stuttering is too variable to demonstrate any significant, non-biological pattern overlooks the complexity of factors influencing the frequency of non-fluency both in the speech of people who are described as stutterers and those who are not considered to have a fluency problem. Young (1985) reviewed many studies in which the speech of stutterers was examined under a number of different conditions. He concluded that the variability of stuttering was predictably influenced by the rate, complexity, content and function of the speech which was produced. These factors suggest the need for a broader-based investigation of constraints upon fluency; in particular, a re-evaluation of the relationship between language processing, language structure and language function and speech fluency.

The role of psycholinguistics

Although our knowledge of the processes involved in normal speech production is limited, there is a growing interest in examining those aspects of linguistic output which transformational grammarians considered to be performance phenomena and therefore 'grammatically irrelevant' (Chomsky and Halle, 1968, 1.3). Studies of the performance behaviour of normal speakers (e.g. Goldman-Eisler, 1968; Fromkin, 1973; Garrett, 1980) and speakers with known language pathology, such as aphasia (Saffran, Schwartz and Martin, 1980) and phonological disorder (Ragsdale and Sisterhen, 1984), have given insights into the way in which language is encoded and decoded. Psycholinguistic studies such as these are concerned not simply with a speaker's abstract linguistic knowledge, but with the processes people employ to produce and perceive spoken and written language. In particular the fluency of normal speakers' performance behaviour has been examined in developmental studies (e.g. Kowal, O'Donnell and Sabine, 1975) and in studies of the form and distribution of fluency disruptions (see for example Goldman-Eisler, 1968; Butterworth, 1980; Beattie, 1983). Starkweather (1980, 1982) has attempted to relate the findings from studies such as these to stuttered speech. In addition there is a growing number of studies applying the psycholinguistic methodology of pausology to the performance behaviour of people who stutter. Because of the breakdown in normal phonetic and prosodic encoding of speech by the person who stutters, phonetic rather than linguistic theory has played the major role in the linguistic study of stuttering. Over ten years ago, however, Eisenson (1975) argued that we should not neglect the linguistic knowledge possessed by a speaker which might underlie disturbances in phonetic and prosodic execution.

The classification of stuttering behaviour has been in use for many years, though it is only in recent years that the influence of psycholinguistic research has led people investigating stuttered speech to look more closely at the total discontinuity behaviour (Love and Jeffress, 1971; Wingate, 1984). The classification of stuttering used by Johnson (1959), for example, was allied to a methodology which would not be considered sound today: he and his colleagues used parental interviews rather than empirical investigations of the speech of young children. When McDearmon (1968) re-evaluated Johnson's data he showed that a significantly larger proportion (63 per cent) of children regarded by their parents as stutterers had simple repetitions and prolongations of sounds in their speech. McDearmon maintained, therefore, that there is a qualitatively different sort of non-fluency in the children who develop stuttering. This has proved not to be an isolated finding but one of the cornerstones of differential diagnosis in young non-fluent children (e.g. Adams, 1977; 1980; Gregory and Hill, 1980; Gregory, 1985; Riley and Riley, 1983).

The implications of breaks in fluency for the speech of non-stutterers has been studied for some years. Goldman-Eisler (1968), for example, reviewed a body of research by herself and her colleagues into — in particular — silent or unfilled pauses (UP) in the speech of normal adult speakers. She argued that UPs occur at predictable places within speech, and indicate not only pausing for breath but pausing in order to plan forthcoming utterances or make lexical selections. Along with Boomer and Dittman (1962), Boomer (1965), and Barik (1968) Goldman-Eisler observed that the locations of UPs and filled pauses (FP) such as 'er', 'um', 'ah' occur at points in the speech output which suggest they play a significant role in the linguistic encoding of an utterance. It was observed that these discontinuities varied according to the complexity of the utterance, although whether the complexity is syntactic or semantic is difficult to decide (see Rochester, 1973, for discussion). Broen and Siegel (1972), however, observed that most adults can manipulate to some extent the occurrence of discontinuities in order, they hypothesised, to enable them to reduce the amount of non-fluency in situations in which the speaker feels more fluency is desirable. They also observed that the ability to exercise control over the degree of fluency was related to the amount of fluency demonstrated by the speaker in non-anxiety-provoking speech situations. There are then some adults who are not regarded as stutterers but who have specific difficulty in inhibiting the amount of discontinuity in their speech. Perhaps for these speakers the non-fluency is functional in a way which makes it difficult to overide.

Functional aspects of other types of discontinuity besides UPs and FPs have been suggested by Heike (1981). On the basis of the analysis of spontaneous speech he has proposed that speakers exert themselves in order to maintain the 'well-formedness' of speech. In order to maintain this quality speakers tend to correct, rather than ignore, errors such as mispronouncing a word, producing a slip of the tongue, or producing a sentence which fails to express the intended idea. However, the correction process itself involves a degree of discontinuity of speech as the speaker moves from forward flow to backtracking and repetition in order to correct the error. Therefore:

Not only are hesitations a normal component of fluency if they occur in moderation, but now pauses and other hesitations can actually be considered as wellformedness phenomena rather than disfluencies, at least as far as they serve as devices by the speaker to produce more error free, high quality speech (Heike, 1981, p. 150).

This observation may suggest reasons for the apparently non-functional behaviour of some adults who, during or even following a moment of stuttering, reiterate the whole utterance which contained the stutter. In Heike's terms the repetition constitutes a repair of the moment of non-fluency by creating a bridge between the start and end of the utterance. In normal speech the process is generally undetectable. In stuttered speech bridging is functionally far less successful but may be retained by some speakers because of the need they perceive to repair fluency. This type of analysis is far removed from the listing of sound types and word classes of stuttered words which formed the basis of 'linguistic' investigations of stuttering until relatively recently (see St Louis, 1979, for a review of these studies). Hamre (1985) describes these locus of stuttering studies as constrained by a too simplistic view of linguistics. Just as the studies of speech discontinuities took little account of the significance of different types of non-fluency and their potential relationship to linguistic encoding, so the locus studies failed to take the linguistic context of stutters into account. Thus the observations made in these studies need not be interpreted as components of the psychological salience of stuttered words (Brown, 1945), they can be explained more systematically in relation to the stress pattern of an utterance (Wingate, 1976, 1985). For example, content words are likely to be longer words, less predictable words and therefore words which will receive a greater degree of stress. Stuttering therefore occurs because of the complex neuromuscular demands made as a result of the need to co-ordinate various physiological mechanisms in order to produce a stressed syllable. As we shall see, the linguistic demands may not be restricted to those involved in the phonetic execution of an utterance.

DEVELOPMENTAL LINGUISTICS AND STUTTERING

After commenting on the development of normal non-fluency in children three types of study will be examined in this section. In the first the fluency and language complexity in non-stuttering children are considered. This comparison leads to the inference that greater linguistic complexity tends to lead to greater amounts of non-fluency though the intersubject variability is high. Nevertheless, the presence of some relationship does suggest that children with language learning problems would be likely to exhibit more non-fluency than children with normal language development. This suggestion will be considered in the second section. Finally the language skills of children with diagnosed fluency problems will be considered.

Starkweather (1980, 1982) addresses the functional significance of non-fluency in non-stuttering children in an attempt to distinguish more precisely between normal and atypical fluency. He suggests that discontinuities are an inevitable component in speech encoding if other aspects of speech which contribute significantly to the impression of fluency, namely high rate and minimal speech effort, are to be preserved. Starkweather observes that while the rate of occurrence of speech discontinuities remains remarkably consistent during language development their form tends to become more sophisticated. In particular, simple repetitive non-fluencies, especially repetitions of parts of words, become much less common than linguistically more advanced forms such as parenthetical remarks like 'I mean ...', 'rather', 'so to say'. Starkweather suggests that children who stutter may not be as effective as normal speakers in using time occupied by discontinuities of one sort or another. Therefore some speakers may need more discontinuities in order to produce speech without an excessive amount of cognitive effort (Starkweather, 1980). What remains to be established is to what extent atypical pause time reflects problems in cognitive–linguistic planning, and at what level or levels of language encoding the putative problems exist.

Language skills and fluency in non-stuttering children

Employing a sentence imitation and/or sentence modelling paradigm Haynes and Hood (1978), Pearl and Bernthal (1980)

57

and Gordon, Luper and Peterson (1986) have all observed a positive relationship between sentence complexity and the amount of non-fluency. Sentence modelling in particular reveals a close relationship between complexity and fluency (Gordon *et al.*, 1986) and these authors found that the 16 five-year-old subjects showed 'highly individual patterns of the disfluency/ complexity relationship' (p. 161). Haynes and Hood (1978) also observed considerable intersubject variability. This appears to be characteristic of all these types of investigation, suggesting, as one might expect, very variable levels of ability in individuals who nevertheless demonstrate recognisable patterns in their performance.

Investigations of the relationship between complexity and fluency in spontaneous speech have been conducted by Colburn and Mysak (1982) and, more recently, by DeJoy and Gregory (1985), who also review three other studies — Haynes and Hood (1977), Wexler and Mysak (1982) and Yairi (1981). All of these studies reveal the individual variability as mentioned above, but a relationship between linguistic complexity and non-fluency was also evident. DeJoy and Gregory (1985), in a large scale ($N=60$) study of two groups of non-stuttering boys in two age groups (3;3–3;9 and 4;9–5;3), observed the development of more adult-like non-fluencies in the younger group. In particular there was an increase in the number of UPs as compared to other types of non-fluency such as part word repetitions, whole word repetitions, phrase repetitions, incomplete phrases, and dysrhythmic phonation. DeJoy and Gregory made the further observation that the increase in UPs was directly linked to increases in the length and complexity of the older children's utterances. There were more pauses at grammatical boundaries in the older group, which the authors suggest 'reflects an increase in the older children's use of compound and/or complex sentences' (DeJoy and Gregory, 1985, p. 114).

Comparison between DeJoy and Gregory's findings and those of the other studies they review reveals some differences which, DeJoy and Gregory suggest, may be partly methodological, and partly because some studies may show an increase in disfluencies at certain ages as the children within their sample 'push their encoding abilities' (p. 119). Colburn and Mysak's (1982) investigation of non-fluencies in the spontaneous speech of preschool children shows good general agreement with the above studies. They also observed that children with the highest syntactic abilities showed a relatively higher degree of phrase-level non-fluency. An apparent contradiction to this observation is offered by Muma (1971), who made a transformational analysis of the spontaneous utterances of 26 four-year-old non-stuttering children. He observed that those children who were the least fluent tended to use the simplest sentences. This could be interpreted as revealing lower than average cognitive–linguistic skills in these children. They produced their speech with greater cognitive effort in which relatively more non-fluency was necessary in order to produce linguistically less complex utterances. These children showed relatively poor cognitive–linguistic abilities but the amount of non-fluency required was nevertheless within normal limits.

An earlier study by Davis (1940) used a simpler analysis of the linguistic complexity of the spontaneous speech of 62 non-stuttering children between two and five years. Davis was able to identify a very slight negative correlation (−0.56) between all repetitions and mean length of response. She was unable to conclude that there was any lack of linguistic development which could explain the incidences of non-fluency. However, in Davis' previous paper (Davis, 1939) she examined the same population and was able to identify significant differences in the amount of non-fluency depending upon the communicative demands of the situation. She observed greatest amounts of non-fluency when children had to direct other children, change activities when instructed to do so by the teacher and when rebutting challenges by other children. Silverman, in a series of papers, explored various aspects of the linguistic performance of ten four-year-old non-stuttering boys. In Silverman (1972) she reported that the more formal situation of an interview elicited greater amounts of non-fluency than were observed in class-room peer interactions. She also noted (Silverman, 1973) that, when talking to themselves, there was more non-fluency in conversations with themselves when their conversation consisted of a dialogue with an imaginary second person. Bjerkan's (1980) larger-scale ($N=110$) study of Norwegian nursery school children (two to six years old) also showed contextual constraints upon fluency. There was, for example, a greater incidence of repetition when speakers had to make a particular effort to gain listener attention. It is clear then that context imposes extra demands on the normal speaker's ability to encode language; the relationship between structural and functional aspects of language will be discussed later.

The fluency of children with speech–language problems

In groups of children with known speech and language difficulty there is some indication that the amount of non-fluency in those groups is higher than in other children. Ragsdale and Sisterhen (1984) investigated the non-fluencies in the spontaneous speech of 40 children between five and six years old who were divided into two groups: articulatory defective and normal. They observed that the experimental group used more UPs, part word repetitions, incomplete sentences, sentence revisions and omissions than the normal group. This finding has been largely replicated in an unpublished study by Urwin (1987). Most other studies which suggest a relationship between linguistic deficiency and fluency have been examinations of the effect of language therapy, and hence presumably accelerated language development upon the fluency of children otherwise regarded as non-stuttering. Hall (1977) reported two case studies in which the number of disfluencies in the speech of two language-delayed children decreased as their linguistic skills developed. Merits-Patterson and Reed (1981), on the other hand, found that of three groups of four to six-year-old children the language-delayed children in therapy showed the greatest rise in the amount of non-fluency as compared to untreated, language-delayed and non language-delayed children. The appearance of non-fluency as language skills develop may be related to the observations by Colburn and Mysak (1982) of four non-stuttering preschool children. The authors found that non-fluency tended to accompany the appearance of new semantic–syntactic constructions in the children's speech.

It has also been observed that there is a higher than average prevalence of atypical non-fluency in the speech of the mentally handicapped (Bloodstein, 1981; Van Riper, 1982; Andrews *et al.*, 1983). In this population of individuals who, as a feature of their handicap, frequently exhibit reduced language skills, the risk of developing a stuttering-like disorder is significantly greater than in the non-mentally handicapped population.

The language skills of children with fluency problems

There is little doubt that many children who stutter also have some degree of speech–language difficulty. In Andrews *et al.* (1983) and Wall and Myers (1984) the majority of studies they reviewed showed that, as a group, children who stutter have a developmental language delay of about six months. Andrews *et al.* (1983) and Bloodstein (1981) conclude that careful examination of the relevant studies suggests that, as a group, stutterers (in the non-mentally handicapped population) tend to have slightly, but significantly, lower IQs than the non-stuttering population. One might speculate that this small difference may be an indication not of the difference in intellectual ability between stutterers and non-stutterers but it may rather indicate a subtle difference in linguistic skills between the two groups. Bloodstein (1981) comments on the relatively few studies which examine the profile of abilities tested. Some studies suggested that stutterers may have had particular difficulties with language-related parts of the assessment batteries. Other investigators did not corroborate these findings but a variety of assessment procedures were used which makes comparison between studies rather difficult.

Turning to the relationship between syntactic complexity and fluency, two studies by Myers and Freeman (1985) on twelve matched four- to six-year-old stuttering and non-stuttering children and by St Louis, Hinzman and Hull (1985) on 72 subjects from six school-age groups, divided into stuttering, cluttering and normal children, suggest there is a positive relationship between increasing syntactic complexity in groups of stuttering children and the frequency with which stutters occur. Such observations in the stuttering population echo the results of studies of non-stuttering children cited earlier, in which aspects of syntatic–semantic and pragmatic constraints tended to be related to fluency. There is no evidence that children who stutter deliberately reduce the complexity of their utterances, and therefore the cognitive effort necessary to encode them. Starkweather (1982) cites some of his earlier work in which he examined comprehension in four- to six-year-old stuttering and non-stuttering children by means of the test for Auditory Comprehension of Language (TACL) (Carrow, 1973) as well as expression by means of mean length of utterance (MLU). Starkweather comments that:

The stutterers produced significantly shorter utterances and significantly lower TACL scores than the non stutterers. Also their TACL scores were positively correlated with their MLU. We concluded that the stutterers were a little slow in acquiring language skills, and it seemed unlikely (although not impossible) that this lag was secondary to stuttering, since it showed up in a comprehension test as well (Stark-weather, 1982, p. 10).

Direct reference to the language problems of children who stutter is made in the therapy programmes of, for example, Riley and Riley (1983), and Wall and Myers (1984). Both are better expressions of multifactorial notions of stuttering onset than the programmes mentioned earlier, in that language, organic and enviromental factors are taken into account in the assessment and treatment of young stutterers. In Riley and Riley's (1983) study of 54 children they assessed and treated, they observed that 75 per cent of pre-six-year-old children improved their fluency without any direct work upon their speech. Therapy may have been directed at improving language skills in some but not all of these, while others may have had therapy directed at manipulating the child's environment in some way. Ninety-one per cent of the older children required specific speech techniques (e.g. prolonged speech — Ingham, 1984) in order to improve fluency. Wall and Myers (1984) have also developed assessment and treatment strategies which aim to examine and, if necessary, offer therapy for their young clients' language development. These authors also point to the success of a number of therapy programmes which achieve fluent speech, particularly in young clients, through the systematic increase in the amount and complexity of language demanded of the client (e.g. Gregory and Hill, 1980; Ryan and Van Kirk, 1978; Shine, 1980; Stocker, 1980). Wall and Myers (1984) point out a number of the cognitive and linguistic components which are involved in the apparently simple task of lengthening an utterance, e.g. increasing semantic and syntactic complexity; increasing sequencing difficulties; and increasing demands upon attention, memory and self-monitoring. These programmes are therefore probably indirectly developing language encoding skills, and are a further indication of the significance of language variables in understanding and treating stuttering.

Homzie and Lindsay (1984), in a recent, wide-ranging review of language and fluency, found the evidence of language problems in children who stutter sufficiently convincing to be able to conclude that: 'the clinician in the field has not been fully aware of the extent to which even the highly intelligent young stutterer may have a basic language problem' (p. 249). The difficulty for the clinician may be in identifying the type of language problem which the stuttererer — of whatever age — may have. The problem is inevitably going to be more subtle than the obvious speech–language problems normally dealt with by the therapist. The extent to which the various levels of language processing interact in the production of normal speech is complex; therefore it is premature to make assumptions about the adequacy for linguistic processing in the speech of people whose only problem is apparently at the phonetic and prosodic level of execution. While it may have considerable face validity — for stutterer and therapist alike — to consider stuttering exclusively as a speech problem, the evidence already cited suggests that the lack of fluency may refect more than a problem in the temporal execution of speech sounds.

FLUENCY AND LEVELS OF LINGUISTIC PROCESSING

In the following sections I will discuss the observations which have been made about fluency and linguistic ability at different levels of linguistic encoding. This will encompass the relationship between stuttering and segmental phonetics and prosody; abstract levels of linguistic representation such as syntax and semantics; and the functional use of language. The main thesis behind this review is similar to that made by Homzie and Lindsay (1984), who maintained, on the basis of their examination of problems in childhood that 'language deficits are an initial contributory factor and a continuing component of the problem [of stuttering]' (p. 248). Of particular interest in subsequent sections will be the way in which it may be possible to understand how linguistic factors might account for the difficulties many stutterers experience in overcoming their speech problem. At this stage, however, we will attempt to show how stutterers of all ages may have complex but subtle language deficits. If this is the case the relationships between the beginning and the developed stutter may become easier to recognise.

There may be a difference in the balance of factors influencing fluency in these groups, but the factors themselves are similar. This view would have repercussions on the assessment and treatment of stutterers, as well perhaps as upon views of what constitutes a successful therapeutic outcome.

Phonetics and stuttering

Considerable attention has been paid to the motor control of speech by stutterers. Adams (1985) reviews a great deal of evidence which suggests that people who stutter experience difficulty in co-ordinating laryngeal and supralaryngeal activity. This occurs not only during moments of stuttering, because motor disco-ordination can also be observed instrumentally in the perceptually fluent speech of the stuttering subjects. As children who do not develop stutters mature, individual speech sounds are produced more rapidly and with reduced variation in length while, at the same time, there is a development in anticipatory coarticulation (Thompson and Hixon, 1979; Kent and Forner, 1980). Evidence for the breakdown in the development of articulatory co-ordination in children who subsequently exhibit confirmed stutters was offered over 20 years ago in the frequently cited study by Stromsta (1965). He analysed spectrograms of the fluent speech of preschool children, all of whom had been labelled as stutterers by their parents. His major finding was that the children who, as a result of abnormal transitions between phonemes and abnormal terminations of phonation within phonemes, had shown failures in coarticulation, were the ones most likely to still be stuttering ten years later. It is generally assumed that this observation offers support for the onset of stuttering is related to an underlying neuromotor disco-ordination. A more recent acoustic analysis by Zebrowski, Conture and Cudahy (1985) of the fluent speech of eleven preschool stutterers and their controls revealed that there were subtle differences in the temporal organisation of the speech of the experimental group. These differences amounted to a relative lack of co-ordination between supraglottal and laryngeal structures when compared to the non-stuttering controls. The authors also felt their study supported other studies of the acoustic structure of the speech of adult stutterers (e.g. Klich and May, 1982) which suggest that there are observable differences in the acoustic structure of the speech of stutterers and non-stutterers.

Prosody and stuttering

Atypical timing in the interrelations of articulator movement have also been observed by Zimmerman (1980) in a video fluorographic study of fluent utterances produced by stuttering subjects. This degree of variability has been observed at the suprasegmental level too. Cooper and Allen (1977), and Bergman (1986), found significantly greater variability of the timing between stressed syllables in stuttering subjects than in non-stuttering controls. Bergman attributes this to the difficulties stutterers may have in the execution of appropriate stress patterns, which he regards as evidence of the motoric difficulties of stutterers. However, although the evidence so far presented has been interpreted as supporting the hypothesis that stutterers have a physiological problem in the timing of the co-ordinated movements required for speech there may be grounds for questioning the separation of cognitive–linguistic planning and motor execution of speech.

Evidence for language encoding difficulties

Love and Jeffress (1971) examined all the fluency disturbances in the speech of adult stutterers and observed that there were more brief UPs in the speech of stuttering adults than in the spontaneous speech of non-stutterers. This finding has been corroborated by Wingate (1984), who examined the spontaneous speech of 20 matched young adult stutterers and non-stutterers. He observed that the stutterers, apart from having more discontinuities of all kinds in their speech than their controls, exhibited a characteristic pattern of discontinuities which, he concluded, showed that stutterers required 'more time ... to resolve whatever decision was necessary to proceed in the lexical sequence' (pp. 233–4). These adult stutterers therefore exhibited some difficulty in planning the sentence structure and/or content, and therefore their surface non-fluency was indicative of a linguistic rather than simply a phonetic or prosodic problem. Winkler and Ramig (1986) investigated

65

the effects of language complexity upon UPs and other temporal phenomena in the speech of nine child stutterers (six to twelve years old) and a control group of nine non-stuttering children. Their results showed that stutterers had more UPs than the control group and the interword pause durations were longer for the experimental group. These differences were apparent in the complex speech task which was essentially spontaneous speech. After considering the results in the light of current theories of stuttering Winkler and Ramig propose a further hypothesis; namely 'that stutterers possess a subtle concomitant language formulation deficit' (p. 226). They cite anecdotal evidence of stutterers (though it is not clear if they refer to their experimental subjects): 'In informal discussions with several stutterers, many have related difficulties with correct word order while speaking as well as uneasiness regarding whether their utterances make sense' (p. 226). The authors felt that the increased UPs may have been necessary in order to provide extra time for language encoding. Although it is difficult to ascertain whether non-fluencies are linked to semantic or syntactic planning they nevertheless appear to indicate the efficiency of language encoding in any given speaker. What is difficult to resolve is whether the pausing in stuttering subjects is required simply to provide extra time for co-ordinating motor skills or whether it is used to organise language more centrally.

The linguistic abilities of adult stutterers have not been subjected to such close scrutiny as the language of children who stutter, possibly because adults frequently report that their only problem is their inability to say what they want to say, rather than in formulating what they want to say. Any problems which are experienced by adults in encoding or decoding language are likely to be subtle, and it is therefore unlikely to be an obvious target for therapy in the same way that it is with young children. Indeed, the effectiveness of therapy directed at speech modification has been shown by a number of authors (see Andrews *et al.*, 1983; Ingham, 1985). Many of these employ some form of rate reduction, at least in the early stages of therapy. This can be argued as necessary from a number of points of view. For example the slower speed should enable co-ordination between phonation and articulation to be established more easily. However this need not be the sole purpose of rate control; slower speech also permits speakers to engage in speech planning for a relatively longer time. It was highlighted in the introduction, however, that many adult stutterers who have developed fluency often find it difficult to maintain (Martin, 1981). It would be very difficult, if indeed at all possible, to decide whether the problems in fluency maintenance are the result of persisting coordination problems, poor acceptance of the new speech form or of themselves as fluent speakers, or of residual difficulties in language encoding resulting from the reduced pause time within the fluent speech. Explanations for the problem of acquired fluency maintenance have employed a number of different theoretical standpoints, but our understanding of the long-term constraints upon fluency, either in normal or clinical populations, is not sufficiently sophisticated either to account for or to help alleviate fluency breakdowns in all clients. Our methods of dealing with fluency breakdowns at whatever stage in therapy may therefore fail to take account of the complexity of the speech production process by focusing upon its motoric components.

The influence of utterance complexity, and the context in which an utterance is produced, have long been observed to form a component of the clinical picture of stuttering in adults as well as children (Bloodstein, 1981; Van Riper, 1982). What is less easy to decide is whether the complexity and contextual factors exacerbate pre-existing difficulties in organising motor behaviour. Evidence for the effect of syntactic complexity comes from studies such as those of Tornick and Bloodstein (1976) and Jayaram (1984). These show that stuttering is more likely to occur at the beginnings of clauses which, as Wall and Myers (1982; p. 443) point out, are locations in utterances where 'a complex arrangement of psycholinguistic and physiological phenomena [occur] ... which, if normally carried out, contribute to fluency'. What is less clear is whether there is increased likelihood of stuttering on more complex clauses regardless of their position in the entire utterance. Jayaram (1984) suggests this may indeed occur, but analysis of spontaneous speech is required.

While the suggestion of linguistic disability forming some component of the stuttering problem is not novel, and appears to have some merit, we still need to understand how a cognitive–linguistic deficit could become a communicative deficit: how might deficits in language structure be related to language function? So far we have suggested that there is considerable overlap in the processes which are involved in the encoding and execution of speech. Might not this overlap extend to other levels of linguistic organisation? This has already been hinted in the suggestion that stutterers may attempt to conform to principles of well-formedness (Heike, 1981) in their speech. In addition, in research conducted by Eisenson and Horowitz (1945) it was observed that decreasing the meaningfulness (or propositionality in their terminology) of a reading task decreased the likelihood of stutters occuring. The level of linguistic organisation implicated in the occurrence of stuttering is that of pragmatics or language function. In effect it is being suggested that a stutterer's attempts to overcome his/her structural linguistic deficits are influenced by the perceived need to communicate. In the final section of this chapter the development of communication management strategies is discussed in relation to the maintenance of stuttering in adulthood.

STUTTERING AS A COMMUNICATION PROBLEM

As children develop, they not only acquire more knowledge of the semantic, syntactic, phonological and phonetic structure of language, they also become aware of the way in which people interact. As well as needing to know the structural rules of a language, children need to learn how to apply those rules. Some part of this knowledge will involve learning how to respond to a speaker's verbal and non-verbal cues in order to facilitate the smooth flow of conversation between speakers. Of particular importance is the management of speaker turns, where one speaker finishes talking and the next begins (McLaughlin, 1984). In order to study the relevance of turn-taking rules (e.g. Duncan, 1972; Sacks, Schegloff and Jefferson, 1974) the speech of stutterers in natural conversation must be examined. Even fairly rudimentary analysis (Duckworth, 1985) shows that stutterers adopt strategies which are commonly found in the speech of non-stutterers and which the stutterer employs for the same purposes but much less successfully. For example many speakers systematically use parenthetical remarks (Starkweather, 1980) and initiators (Quirk and Greenbaum, 1973) (e.g. 'well', 'er' and other FPs) in order to maintain the conversational turn while momentarily not contributing substantially to the conversational content (McClay and Osgood, 1959).

Stutterers may be eager to prevent breaks in continuity such as might occur at the start of a conversational turn, or to repair breaks during conversation because the stutterer may perceive these breaks in speech flow as turn-taking cues. The failure to initiate or proceed with an utterance may therefore be equated with the loss of conversational turn by the stutterer. What seems likely to outweigh the significance of any difficulties a stutterer might experience in organising an utterance in a conversation is his/her desire to hold the conversational turn. Adult speakers recognise the need to signal their intention to begin or continue talking even before they have fully organised a response. Even if the adult stutterer does have relatively more difficulty in organising a response than the non-stutterer, this does not mean that the usual turn-taking and floor-holding rules will be relaxed by the stutterer, undoubtedly because he/she is aware that relaxation on his/her part is likely to lead to a loss of conversational turn. In referring to the behaviour of non-stuttering participants in conversations Wardhaugh (1985) comments:

> if you are hesitant, the best course of action for you is to hold on to the floor once you have gained it by almost refusing to acknowledge the presence of others: if you do not see them [by avoiding eye contact], in one sense they are not there to interrupt you, they must use more than their eyes to gain access to the floor — they must actually interrupt you and appear somewhat rude in doing so (p. 87).

If stutterers do reduce gaze — and there is ample clinical evidence that they do (e.g. Sheehan, 1970) — and if they do employ initiators and bridging devices to maintain the integrity of their conversational turn they are manipulating communication rules in order to assist them in overcoming problems which may occur at a different level in linguistic planning. This may also lead to a manipulation of utterance content which, as has been suggested, can play a significant part in influencing cognitive–linguistic difficulty. These manipulations may in fact be made not because of real encoding difficulties but because the speaker, perhaps on the basis of past experience, believes he/she will experience difficulty. The speaker may therefore produce utterances of minimal content which may or may not be stuttered: the — real or perceived — difficulty in planning leading to the manipulation of interactions. The manipulation itself, however, reduces yet further the time the speaker can spend on organising the utterance so any linguistic encoding difficulty may be exacerbated rather than helped as the speaker concentrates greater energy on the form of the utterance at the expense of its content. The linguistic breakdown described here is at the functional level of interpersonal communication, but because the 'levels' are interrelated it cannot be assumed that a stutterer's syntactic, semantic and pragmatic abilities are unexceptional.

Interactions between stutterers and non-stutterers

Recent studies of interactions between stutterers and non-stutterers suggest how stutterers may develop an awareness of the functional inadequacy of their speech and therefore attempt to compensate for this. Myers and Freeman (1985) conducted a video analysis of mothers of stuttering and non-stuttering four-to six-year-old children during play sessions with their own and with other children. They noted the tendency for all mothers to interrupt non-fluent speech more than fluent speech. Stutters may be misperceived as turn-taking signals, and consequently stutterers may feel they should avoid such signals and thus develop strategies for avoiding breaks in the forward flow of speech. An incidental result of interactional research of this type may be to re-emphasise the importance of parent–child interactions. Despite the reduction in influence of the Johnsonian model of stuttering onset speech therapists, when canvassed for their opinions about stuttering and stuttering therapy (Cooper and Cooper, 1985; Cooper and Rustin, 1985), reveal that they feel it is still important to consider both the child and his/her environment. In the past, positive parent–child interactions have been encouraged and guidelines set out in booklet form (e.g. Ainsworth and Frazer-Gruss, 1977). These tend to focus on environmental manipulations which are believed to reduce pressure on the child to compete verbally, and therefore make the child less likely to stutter. Zwitman's (1978) programme of parental involvement goes further than encouraging good parenting practices, and encourages both parents and children to reduce their speech rate. In recent years the significance of parental and child speech rate reduction has been stressed by an increasing number of writers who have also provided empirical support for this practice (e.g. Shine, 1980;

Johnson, 1980; Gregory and Hill, 1980; Ingham, 1983).

There have, until recently, been fewer studies of the way in which between parents and stuttering children interact. The value of encouraging changes in interactional style between parents and stuttering children has therefore lacked a theoretical framework other than appealing to principles of good child-rearing practice, and has been criticised because of this (Ingham, 1984). What has been overlooked is how the inappropriate adult interactions have developed, and to what extent they are functional and resistant to change. The difficulty of maintaining fluent speech in later life may be related less to the mechanical difficulty of producing fluent speech than to the — real or perceived — demands fluency places upon the process of language encoding.

Studies of interactional patterns and the development of functional communication in children who stutter may ultimately indicate that (some) stutterers develop inappropriate communication strategies which may have aimed to conceal cognitive–linguistic deficits. Strategies such as repeating words and phrases or using frequent filler words may persist because speakers use them to overcome whatever breaks in fluency are perceived. The maladaptive nature of these strategies often outweighs any superficial fluency gains, but the perceived gain may be considerable and may therefore perpetuate their continued use. Adults tend to describe the precipitation of stuttering in terms of responses to some combination of speech sounds (or initial 'letters'), words or situations. Indeed, it is difficult to separate the effects of the speaker's expectation of difficulty from involuntary breaks in fluency. The evidence already adduced demonstrates that, however appealing neuromuscular explanations of stuttering behaviour are, instances of stuttering may relate more to the structure and function of language than to its motoric execution. The examination of these non-phonetic components of stuttering in adults has probably received less attention because its motoric manifestations are so much more evident, and are so immediately responsive to therapy. Given the apparent normality of language functioning in many stutterers on at least some occasions, the deficit may simply create for the adult stutterers the context in which they feel themselves more likely to stutter, and therefore make them more likely to manipulate their utterances.

The mismanagement of interactions by adult stutterers has

been examined in at least one study. Jensen, Markel and Beverung (1986) manipulated dyadic encounters between nine adult stutterers and a non-stuttering accomplice. The subjects showed three behaviours which inhibited the production of fluent speech and adversely affected conversational management. Firstly, at conversational turns they tended to respond much faster than non-stutterers. Severe stutterers in particular exhibited a less than normal pause time at conversational turns. Such rapidity will not be likely to promote the smooth co-ordination of cognitive–linguistic and physiological components of speech. If there is some sort of cognitive–linguistic deficit in adults who stutter a rapid response will reduce the amount of available planning time which, in turn, makes the likelihood of fluency breakdown even greater. The second finding in Jensen *et al*'s study shows that stutterers may fail to employ strategies conventionally found in conversational exchanges. Turntaking information is communicated through verbal and non-verbal channels (Beattie, 1980, 1983) but Jensen *et al.* (1986) found that stutterers tended to use less eye contact before and after making a response than non-stutterers. Research by Argyle, Lefebvre and Cook (1974) revealed that listeners do not like minimal gaze, perhaps because, as Wardaugh (1985) suggests, it may be used as a strategy to prevent interruption. Repeated gaze aversion, however useful it might be for enhancing a stutterer's speech management, may therefore lead to a disruption in communication between the stutterer and the listener. Jensen *et al.*'s third observation was that the stuttering subjects failed to give appropriate body movement signals. Duncan (1972), and Beattie (1983) have observed the effect gesture can have on preventing a listener from taking over the conversation even during a moment of silence. Secondary movements which often form a part of stuttering behaviour (Bloodstein, 1981; Van Riper, 1982) are, often gross, movements of limbs, trunk or face which appear to be connected with the release of a stutter. However, close inspection of normal non-fluencies and body movements has revealed that the latter tend to accompany the resolution of the non-fluency as if the movement provided a means of dissipating energy expended in overcoming the discontinuity (Hadar, Steiner and Rose, 1984). The stutterer may use such movements in a similar manner to a non-stutterer even though the movements are quantitatively greater. However, before a stutterer overcomes a fluency break, Jensen *et al.*'s (1986) observation suggests that the normal body motion signals to the listener may not occur. They noted that there was relatively less body movement by stutterers during moments of stuttering than in the non-stutterers during their non-fluencies. This, they suggested, may give the listener the wrong clues about the intentions of the stutterer to hold the floor.

There is need for further analysis of stuttering in adults as well as in children outside the well-tried and tested frameworks of reading and within more naturalistic conversational settings. In this way the interpretation of stuttering as primarily a speech disorder may need to be revised. My own investigation of three adult stutterer and non-stutterer conversational dyads suggested that the occurrence of stuttering could be linked to the degree of demand placed upon stutterers within the conversational exchange (Duckworth, 1985). Fluency, or the lack of it, was related to the function of the stutterers' contributions. Stuttering was frequently linked to responses made to *wh* questions, and fluency invariably accompanied those utterances made by the stutterer which encouraged the non-stutterer to continue talking. These are termed back-channel utterances and consist of brief statements expressing interest or reiterating or completing a small portion of the speaker's sentence (McLaghlin, 1984). Responses to *yes–no* questions, and statements not related to questions, were associated with less stuttering than responses to *wh* questions but much more than with back-channel utterances. This observation leads to intriguing questions about the degree to which stutterers and non-stutterers may manipulate conversational interactions in order to promote fluent speech.

The therapeutic significance of the linguistic investigation of stuttering remains to be shown, but focusing exclusively upon the observable motor behaviour has not proved to be an adequate solution for many people who stutter. Linguistic analysis of the problem encourages stuttering to be viewed in terms of communication as a whole, rather than as a fragment of the process. Ultimately this broadening of perspective may have more therapeutic significance than the creation of yet another 'method' for treating the stutterer.

REFERENCES

Adams, M.R. (1977) A clinical strategy for differentiating the normally nonfluent child and the incipient stutterer. *Journal of Fluency Disorders, 2*, 141-8

Adams, M.R. (1980) The young stutterers; diagnosis, treatment and assessment of progress. *Seminars in Speech, Language and Hearing, 1*, 289-99

Adams, M.R. (1985) The speech physiology of stutterers: present status. *Seminars in Speech and Language, 6*, 177-90

Ainsworth, S. and Fraser-Gruss, J. (1977) *If your child stutters: a guide for parents*, Speech Foundation of America, Memphis

Andrews, G., Craig, A., Feyer, A.M., Hoddinott, S., Howie, P. and Neilson, M. (1983) Stuttering; a review of research findings circa 1982. *Journal of Speech and Hearing Disorders, 48*, 226-46

Argyle, M., Lefebvre, L. and Cook, M. (1974) The meaning of five patterns of gaze. *European Journal of Social Psychology, 4*, 126-36

Barik, H.C. (1968) On defining juncture pauses: a note on Boomer's 'Hesitation and grammatical encoding'. *Language and Speech, 11*, 156-9

Beattie, G.W. (1980) The role of language production processes in the organisation of behaviour in face-to-face interaction. In B. Butterworth, (ed.), *Language production*, vol. 1: *Speech and talk*. Academic Press, London

Beattie, G.W. (1983) *Talk: an analysis of speech and non-verbal behaviour in conversation*. Open University Press, Milton Keynes

Bergman, G. (1986) Studies in stuttering as a prosodic disturbance. *Journal of Speech and Hearing Disorders, 29*, 290-300

Bjerkan, B. (1980) Word fragmentations and repetitions in the spontaneous speech of 2–6 year old children. *Journal of Fluency Disorders, 5*, 137-48

Bloodstein, O. (1981) *A handbook on stuttering*, 3rd edn, National Easter Seal Society, Chicago

Boberg, E., Yeudall, L.T., Schopflocher, D. and Bo-Lassen, P. (1983) The effect of an intensive behavioral program on the distribution of EEG alpha powers in stutterers during the processing of verbal and visuospatial information. *Journal of Fluency Disorders, 8*, 245-64

Boomer, D.S. (1965) Hesitation and grammatical encoding. *Language and Speech, 8*, 148-58

Boomer, D.S. and Dittman, A.T. (1962) Hesitation pauses and juncture pauses in speech, *Language and Speech, 5*, 215-20

Broen, P.A. and Siegel, G.M. (1972) Variations in normal speech disfluencies. *Language and Speech, 15*, 219-31

Brown, S.F. (1945) The loci of stuttering in the speech sequence. *Journal of Speech Disorders, 10*, 181-92

Butterworth, B. (1980) Evidence from pauses in speech. In B. Butterworth, (ed.), *Language production*, vol. 1: *Speech and talk*, Academic Press, London

Carrow, E. (1973) *Test for auditory comprehension of language*, Teaching Resources Corporation, Boston

Chomsky, N. and Halle, M. (1968) *The sound patterns of English*, Harper & Row, New York

Colburn, N. and Mysak, E. (1982) Development disfluency and emerging grammar. II. Co-occurrence of disfluency with specified semantic–syntactic structures. *Journal of Speech and Hearing Research*, 25, 421-7

Cooper, E.B. (1979) Intervention procedures for the young stutterer. In H.H. Gregory, (ed.), *Controversies about stuttering therapy*, University Park Press, Baltimore

Cooper, E.B. and Cooper, C.S. (1985) Clinician attitudes toward stuttering: a decade of change (1973–1983). *Journal of Fluency Disorders, 10*, 19-34

Cooper, E.B. and Rustin, L. (1985) Clinician attitudes toward stuttering in the United States and Great Britain: a cross cultural study. *Journal of Fluency Disorders, 10*, 19-34

Cooper, M.H. and Allen, G.D. (1977) Timing control accuracy in stutterers. *Journal of Speech and Hearing Research, 20*, 55-71

Davis, D. (1939) The relation of repetitions in the speech of young children to certain measures of language maturity and situational factors. Part I. *Journal of Speech Disorders, 4*, 303-18

Davis, D. (1940) The relation of repetitions in the speech of young children to certain measures of language maturity and situational factors. Parts II and III. *Journal of Speech Disorders, 5*, 235-46

DeJoy, D. and Gregory, H.H. (1985) The relationship between age and frequency of disfluency in preschool children. *Journal of Fluency Disorders, 10*, 107-22

Duckworth, M.S. (1985) Stuttering as a variable in conversation. Paper given at The Oxford Dysfluency Conference, 7–9 August

Duncan, S. (1972) Some signals and rules for taking speaking turns in conversations. *Journal of Personality and Social Psychology, 23*, 283-92

Eisenson, J. (1975) Stuttering as perseverative behaviour. In J. Eisenson, (ed.), *Stuttering: a second symposium*, Harper & Row, New York

Eisenson, J. and Horowitz, E. (1945) The influence of propositionality on stuttering. *Journal of Speech Disorders, 10*, 193-98

Fromkin, V. (1973) *Speech errors as linguistic evidence*, Mouton, The Hague

Garrett, M.F. (1980) Levels of processing in sentence production. In B. Butterworth, (ed.), *Language Production*, vol. 1: *Speech and talk*, Academic Press, London

Goldman-Eisler, F. (1968) *Psycholinguistics: experiments in spontaneous speech*, Academic Press, London

Gordon, P.A., Luper, H. and Peterson, H.A. (1986) The effects of syntactic complexity on the occurrence of disfluencies in 5 year old stutterers. *Journal of Fluency Disorders, 11*, 151-64

Gregory, H.H. (1985) Prevention of stuttering: management of early stages. In R.F. Curlee, and W.H. Perkins, (ed.), *Nature and treatment of stuttering: new directions*, Taylor & Francis, London/College-Hill Press, San Diego

Gregory, H.H. and Hill, D. (1980) Stuttering therapy for children. *Seminars in Speech, Language and Hearing, 1*, 351-62

Hadar, V., Steiner, T.J. and Rose, F.C. (1984) The relationship between head movements and speech disfluencies. *Language and Speech, 27*, 333-42

Hall, P. (1977) The occurrence of disfluency in language disordered school age children. *Journal of Speech and Hearing Disorders, 42*, 364-9

Hamre, C.E. (1985) Stuttering as a cognitive–linguistic disorder. In R.F. Curlee and W.H. Perkins, (eds), *Nature and treatment of stuttering: new directions*. Taylor & Francis, London/College-Hill Press, San Diego

Haynes, W. and Hood, S. (1977) An investigation of linguistic and fluency variables in nonstuttering children from discrete chronological age groups. *Journal of Fluency Disorders, 2*, 57-74

Haynes, W. and Hood, S. (1978) Disfluency changes in children as a function of the systematic modification of linguistic complexity. *Journal of Communication Disorders, 11*, 79-93

Heike, A.E. (1981) A content-processing view of hesitation phenomena. *Language and Speech, 24*, 147-60

Homzie, M.J. and Lindsay, J.S. (1984) Language and the young stutterer; a new look at old theories and findings. *Brain and Language, 22*, 231-52

Ingham, R.J. (1983) Spontaneous remission of stuttering; when will the emperor realise he has no clothes on? In D. Prins, and R.J. Ingham, (eds), *Treatment of stuttering in early childhood*, College-Hill, San Diego

Ingham, R.J. (1984) *Stuttering and behaviour therapy*, Taylor & Francis, London/College-Hill Press, San Diego

Ingham R.J. (1985) Stuttering treatment outcome evaluation: closing the credibility gap. *Seminars in Speech and Language, 6*, 105-24

Ingham, R.J. and Andrews, C. (1973) Details of a token economy stuttering therapy programme for adults. *Australian Journal of Human Communication Disorders, 1*, 13-20

Jayaram, M. (1984) Distribution of stuttering in sentences: relationship to sentence length and clause position. *Journal of Speech and Hearing Research, 27*, 338-41

Jensen, P.L., Markel, N.M. and Beverung, J.W. (1986) Evidence of conversational disrhythmia in stutterers. *Journal of Fluency Disorders, 11*, 183-200

Johnson, L.J. (1980) Facilitating parental involvement in therapy of the disfluent child. *Seminars in Speech, Language and Hearing, 1*, 301-8

Johnson, W. (1959) *The onset of stuttering.* University of Minnesota Press, Minneapolis

Kent, R.D. (1985) Stuttering as a temporal programming disorder. In R.F. Curlee and W.H. Perkins, (eds), *Nature and treatment of stuttering: new directions* Taylor & Francis, London/College-Hill Press, San Diego

Kent, R.D. and Forner, L.L. (1980) Speech segment durations in sentence recitation by children and adults. *Journal of Phonetics, 8*, 157-68

Klich, R.J. and May, G.M. (1982) Spectrographic study of vowels in stutterers' fluent speech. *Journal of Speech and Hearing Research, 25*, 364-70

Kowal, S., O'Donnell, P.C. and Sabine, E.F. (1975) Development of temporal patterning and vocal hesitations in spontaneous narratives. *Journal of Psycholinguistic Research, 4*, 195-207

Love, L.R. and Jeffress, L.A. (1971) Identification of brief pauses in the fluent speech of stutterers and non stutterers. *Journal of Speech and Hearing Research, 14*, 229-40

McClay, H. and Osgood, C.E. (1959) Hesitation phenomena in spontaneous English speech. *Word, 15*, 19-44

McDearmon, J.R. (1968) Primary stuttering at the onset of stuttering: a reexamination of the data. *Journal of Speech and Hearing Research, 11*, 631-7

McLaghlin, M.L. (1984) *Conversation: how talk is organized*, Sage, Beverley Hills

Martin, R.R. (1981) Introduction and perspective; review of published studies. In E. Boberg, (ed.), *Maintenance of fluency: proceedings of the Banff Conference*. Elsevier, New York

Merits-Patterson, R. and Reed, C. (1981) Disfluencies in the speech of language delayed children. *Journal of Speech and Hearing Research, 24*, 55-8

Moore, W.H. (1985) Central nervous characteristics of stutterers. In R.F. Curlee and W.H. Perkins, (eds), *Nature and treatment of stuttering: new directions*. Taylor & Francis, London/College-Hill Press, San Diego

Muma, J.R. (1971) Syntax of preschool fluent and disfluent speech: a transformational analysis. *Journal of Speech and Hearing Research. 14*, 428-41

Myers, S.L. and Freeman, F.J. (1985) Are mothers of stutterers different? An investigation of social communicative interaction. *Journal of Fluency Disorders, 10*, 193-210

Pearl, S. and Bernthal, J. (1980) The effect of grammatical complexity upon disfluency behavior of nonstuttering preschool children. *Journal of Fluency Disorders, 5*, 55-68

Quirk, R. and Greenbaum, S. (1973) *A University Grammar of English*. Longman, London

Ragsdale, J.D. and Sisterhen, D.H. (1984) Hesitation phenomena in the spontaneous speech of normal and articulatory defective children. *Language and Speech, 27*, 235-44

Riley, G.D. and Riley, J. (1983) Evaluation as a basis for intervention. In D. Prins and R.J. Ingham, (eds), *Treatment of stuttering in early childhood: methods and issues*, College-Hill Press, San Diego

Rochester, S.R. (1973) The significance of pauses in spontaneous speech. *Journal of Psycholinguistic Research, 2*, 51-81

Ryan, B. and Van Kirk, B. (1978) *Monterey Fluency Program*. Monterey Learning Systems, Palo Alto, California

Sacks, S.H., Schegloff, E.A. and Jefferson, G.A. (1974) A simplest systematics for the organization of turn taking for conversation. *Language, 50*, 697-735

Saffran, E.M., Schwartz, M.F. and Martin, O.S.M. (1980) Evidence from aphasia: isolating the components of a production model. In B. Butterworth, (ed.), *Language production*, vol. 1: *Speech and talk*. Academic Press, London,

Shames, C.H. and Florance, C.L. (1980) Stutter Free Speech, Charles E. Merrill, Columbus, Ohio

Sheehan, J.G. (1970) *Stuttering: research and therapy*, Harper & Row, New York

Shine, R.E. (1980) Direct management of the beginning stutterer. *Seminars in Speech Language and Hearing, 1*, 339-50

Silverman, E.M. (1972) Generality of disfluency data collected from preschoolers. *Journal of Speech and Hearing Research, 15*, 84-92

Silverman, E.M. (1973) The influence of preschoolers' speech usage on their disfluency frequency. *Journal of Speech and Hearing Research, 16*, 474-81

St Louis, K.O. (1979) Linguistic and motor aspects of stuttering. In N.J. Lass, (ed.), *Speech and language: advances in basic research and practice*, vol. 1, Academic Press, New York

St Louis, K.O., Hinzman, A.R. and Hull, F.M. (1985) Studies of cluttering; disfluency and language measures in young possible clutterers and stutterers. *Journal of Fluency Disorders, 10*, 151-72

Starkweather, C.W. (1980) Speech fluency and its development in normal children. In N.J. Lass, (ed.), *Speech and language: advances in basic research and practice*, Academic press, New York

Starkweather, C.W. (1982) The development of fluency in normal children. In *Stuttering Therapy: Prevention and Intervention with Children*. Proceedings of the 1982 conference, Evaluation of Disfluency, Prevention of Stuttering, and Management of Fluency Problems in Children, at Northwestern University, Speech Foundation of America, Memphis

Stocker, B. (1980) *The Stocker probe technique: for diagnosis and treatment of stuttering in young children*, Modern Education Corporation, Tulsa

Stromsta, C. (1965) A spectrographic study of dysfluencies labelled as stuttering by parents. *De Therapia Vocis et Loquelae*, vol. I; XIII Congress of the International Society of Logopedics and Phonatrics, pp. 317-20

Thompson, A.B. and Hixon, T.J. (1979) Nasal air flow during normal speech production. *Cleft Palate Journal, 16*, 412-30

Tornick, G.B. and Bloodstein, O. (1976) Stuttering and sentence length. *Journal of Speech and Hearing Research, 19*, 651-4

Urwin, R. (1987) Investigating discontinuities in the speech of phonologically disordered children. Unpublished dissertation for BSc(Hons), Speech Therapy, University of Wales

Van Riper, C. (1982) *The nature of stuttering*, 2nd. edn, Prentice-Hall Englewood Cliffs, NJ

Wall, M.J. and Myers, F.L. (1984) *Clinical management of childhood stuttering*, University Park Press, Baltimore

Wardhaugh, R. (1985) *How conversation works*, Blackwell, Oxford

Wexler, R.B. and Mysak, E.D. (1982) Disfluency characteristics of 2-, 4-, and 6-year-old males. *Journal of Fluency Disorders, 7*, 37-46

Wingate, M.E. (1976) *Stuttering: theory and treatment*, Irvington, New York

Wingate, M.E. (1984) Pause loci in stuttered and normal speech. *Journal of Fluency Disorders, 9*, 227-36

Wingate, M.E. (1985) Stuttering as a prosodic disorder. In R.F. Curlee and W.H. Perkins, (eds), *Nature and treatment of stuttering: new directions*, Taylor & Francis, London/College-Hill Press, San Diego

Winkler, L.E. and Ramig, P. (1986) Temporal characteristics in the fluent speech of child stutterers and non stutterers. *Journal of Fluency Disorders, 11*, 217-30

Yairi, E. (1981) Disfluencies of normally speaking two year old children. *Journal of Speech and Hearing Research, 24*, 490-5

Yeudall, L.T. (1985) A neuro-psychological theory of stuttering. *Seminars in Speech and Language, 6*, 197-224

Young, M.A. (1985) Increasing the frequency of stuttering. *Journal of Speech and Hearing Research, 28*, 282-93

Zebrowski, P.M., Conture, E.G. and Cudahy, E.A. (1985) Acoustic analysis of young stutterers' fluency: preliminary observations. *Journal of Fluency Disorders, 10*, 173-92

Zimmermann, G. (1980) Articulatory dynamics of fluent utterances of stutterers and non stutterers. *Journal of Speech and Hearing Research, 23*, 95-107

Zwitman, D.H. (1978) *The disfluent child: a management program*, University Park Press, Baltimore

5

The Role of Linguistics in Psycholinguistic Theory Construction

Andrew Spencer

INTRODUCTION

In this chapter I am concerned with the relationship between one variety of linguistic theory, generative grammar, and psycholinguistic theory. Generative grammar has always been presented by its proponents as a 'psychologically real' grammar, and it has always been held that linguistic theory is a formalised theory of the 'grammatical competence' of a language user, which underlies his language behaviour ('performance'). These notions have provoked a good deal of controversy. I shall assume, however, that the philosophical claims of generative grammarians are roughly true, and pursue the leading ideas of the theory in the context of the development of articulation. To the extent that this can be done without incoherence or contradiction we will have vindication of the generativists' standpoint.

Despite the much-discussed distinction between 'competence' and 'performance', generative grammar is in a certain sense a theory of linguistic performance. However, the performer is an idealised language user whose language behaviour is indistinguishable from the pure working of the abstract grammar written by linguists. This is not to say that the language user exists on some abstract ideal plane distinct from the real world; merely that linguists abstract away from real world variables which the theory is too rudimentary to handle. For some linguists this is no longer a tenable position, and they adopt the view that linguistics is the study of a totally abstract domain in some abstract dimension, rather like mathematics (cf. Katz, 1984 for a philosophical defence of this Platonist theory of linguistics). This is emphatically not the position that, e.g.,

Chomsky espouses, nor the one that I adopt.

The reasons for making such idealisations are simple: without them it is difficult to construct a rich and rigorous theory, free of handwaving. Implicit in this approach is the assumption that once a sufficiently robust theory of linguistics is available some of these ideality assumptions can be dropped or relaxed to bring the theory closer to the real world. In practice, however, there has been comparatively little theory construction in psycholinguistics which has taken this path. Some work on parsing (Kimball, 1973; Frazier and Fodor, 1978) has this character, as does pretty well all work on learnability theory (e.g. Wexler and Culicover, 1980; Pinker, 1984). However, the bulk of psycholinguistics has a somewhat ambivalent relationship to linguistic theory, if not a frankly hostile one.

One area in which linguistic theory has often played a leading role is in articulation development (often misleadingly called 'phonological development'). The two most influential theoretical statements in this field, Jakobson (1968) and Smith (1973), both take linguistic theory as their point of departure and address the problem as a problem in the application of linguistic theory and methodology to a non-standard domain. They relax the usual assumptions respectively of Praguian structuralism and generative phonology only to the extent that this is absolutely required by the data. This is not a universally accepted stance. Locke (1983a) cites with approval a passage from Ferguson and Farwell (1975) in which the latter authors characterise their approach as an attempt 'to understand children's phonological development in itself so as to improve our phonological theory even if this requires new theoretical constructs for the latter' (1975, p. 437). Admittedly, Ferguson and Farwell are addressing the problem of very early development when properly linguistic patterning is not very evident, and it is not entirely clear that non-linguistic determinants of behaviour are not swamping out the linguistic determinants. Nonetheless, the view that linguistic theory should be dependent on psycholinguistic theory rather than the other way around is common (amongst psycholinguists, at least), despite the fact that it flies in the face of the philosophical basis of linguistic theory.

Despite my confident opening remarks, however, it turns out to be very difficult to trace the development of a psycholinguistic theory from its supposedly linguistic roots, even in individual cases. There are a number of reasons for this.

First, although linguistic theory presupposes idealisations, research has to proceed in the real world. In some cases the usual sources of data (native informant judgements) turn out to be equivocal or insufficient, and then other ('external') sources of data might be sought. One of these could be child language. Thus, in principle, psycholinguistic data (which always means, implicitly, psycholinguistic theory) could influence linguistic theory construction. This is not a serious problem, however, because in practice such occurrences will be in the minority and in any case external data of this kind are only important in the absence of strong evidence from customary sources. It is still a mistake to elevate this occasional research strategy to the status of methodological principle.

The second problem is more serious, and concerns the very nature of theory construction and the nature of scientific inquiry. In practice scientific research proceeds in a very 'messy' fashion, and seldom follows the dogmas of philosophers of science. Thus, many important and fruitful research ideas are the result of asking the wrong questions in the wrong way for the wrong reasons. On the other hand if research were to follow some kind of recipe which involved proceeding from the more abstract to the less abstract it would probably grind to a stultifying halt. Therefore, when I say that a psycholinguistic theory must be derived by relaxing ideality assumptions in linguistic theory I am not necessarily saying that this is the way experiments should be conducted. Rather I am talking about the logical status of the theories proposed.

In order to make this view coherent, however, I owe the reader some account of what I mean by a theory (as opposed, for instance, to an occasional model or some other kind of partial theoretical explanation for isolated subdomains). This relates to the question of what constitutes an explanation as opposed to a description of a set of facts. Now, it is perfectly possible to provide a careful description of some set of phenomena and suggest an explanation, outside the bounds of any established theory, for why the data might be so. This, indeed, is the commonest research strategy in a complex area such as psycholinguistics. However, this must not be mistaken for genuine theory construction. Such partial or *ad hoc* explanations are extremely valuable in a variety of ways (applied and theoretical) and I am not suggesting that such activity be curtailed. However, it is also essential to develop a global account of the field with a sound (that is consistent) explanatory basis. It is to this problem that my chapter is addressed.

Discussion of this problem, even within the limited domain of articulation development, would probably require at least a monograph. For the purposes of this chapter, therefore, I have decided to borrow the recent philosophical discussion of theories of language development provided by Atkinson (1982). He sets out five conditions of adequacy on developmental theories which determine their explanatory merit. The conditions are not entirely unproblematical but Atkinson's work provides a very solid basis for evaluation.

The question finally arises of why this is important. In answer to this I can merely say that to me it is intuitively obvious that research is likely to be hindered by conceptual confusion (even if such confusion may occasionally be a fruitful, if adventitious, source of insightful hypotheses). The harmful effects of such confusions are occasionally charted in the literature. I shall briefly discuss some of these and present some thoughts on the nature of 'phonological disability' from the standpoint of the preceding discussion.

In the first section I discuss the idealisations of generative linguistic theory. Section 2 provides a principled way of relaxing the assumption of instantaneous acquisition in a single bound (2.1) and an alternative to the assumption that a language user has just one grammar for all modalities of use. Section 3.1 offers a revision to Smith's (1973) model of articulation development (discussed in much greater detail in Chapter 6). Section 3.2 outlines a very similar theory due to Lise Menn, and presents a criticism of some of its underpinnings on the basis of the discussion of the previous sections. Having presented an interim summary in section 4, I evaluate my theory of development fairly exhaustively in section 5 against the conditions on explanatory theories proposed by Atkinson (1982), concluding immodestly that it fares very well. Section 6 is a discussion of the implications of the previous discussion for research in phonological disability.

1. THE IDEALISATIONS OF LINGUISTIC THEORY

The linguistic theory I shall be assuming is predicated over the following assumptions:

83

(1)   The grammar of a human language is represented in the minds of its users.

(2)   The mentally represented grammar plays a causal role in language behaviour.

(3)   The language user is free from all dysfunction, has infinite memory capacity, infinite extralinguistic knowledge, etc. and his performance is error-free.

(4)   The grammar of any language includes a core component which is universal and hence specified in the genotype.

(5)   The grammar of a particular language is acquired by the learner on the basis of his knowledge of the universal core component (UG); differences in structure between the grammars of different languages are best regarded as parameters.

(6a)   Language acquisition is a function which maps the learner's initial knowledge state (i.e. UG) into a final state (adult knowledge of a particular language) as a result of exposure to a degenerate sampling of utterances in the language (not all of them necessarily well-formed) within a perfectly homogeneous speech community.

(6b)   Language acquisition is instantaneous.[1]

This summary is culled from Chomsky (1965, 1975, 1980, 1981).

Assumptions (1) − (6) do not enjoy the same status in linguistic theory; (1), (2), (4), (5) are actually working hypotheses held to be roughly true, while (3) and (6) are idealisations which are not literally true. This means that while a psycholinguistic theory of normal mature language function is at liberty to take over the former set of assumptions, it is not at liberty to adopt (3) or (6). Assumption (3) rules out any theory of linguistic performance whatsoever, while (6) rules out any non-trivial theory of acquisition, as do assumptions (1) − (3). The most linguistic theory could provide is what is provided by assumptions (4) and (5), viz. a set of 'boundary conditions' on psycholinguistic theory construction.

Let us call a theory adhering to (1) − (6) a 'pure competence theory' and contrast it with a theory whose aim is to explain exhaustively all aspects of real-time language behaviour, a 'pure performance theory'. Between these two extremes there will be indefinitely many intermediate theories, which relax the assumptions of the competence theory while abstracting away from real-world variation covered in the performance theory.[2]

2. PSYCHOLINGUISTIC THEORY CONSTRUCTION

2.1. The course of acquisition

Construction of a psycholinguistic theory could as a matter of logical principle proceed in any of three ways. In the first of these the objective of theory construction is some notional 'complete performance theory'. This is built by abstracting away minimally from some of the variability in the data, and then analysing the data collected within some descriptive framework derived from psychological theory in a non-linguistic cognitive domain. Examples would be theories which approach language learning from, say, a Piagetian viewpoint, 'functionally based' theories and so on. I will call this approach the 'inductive strategy' and the type of theory it gives rise to I shall call a 'psychological psycholinguistic theory'.

The point of departure for the second type is linguistic theory and methodology. Child language data are treated more or less like any linguistic data, and the aim of theory construction in the first instance is the writing of a grammar. Paradigm examples of this style of research in phonological development are Jakobson's (1968) Praguian theory and Smith's (1973) generative theory of development. We may refer to this research style as the 'deductive strategy'. It leads to a theory type I shall call a 'linguistic psycholinguistic theory'.

In practice, of course, a third alternative is generally adopted in which the psycholinguistic theory is forged out of a mixture of psychological theoretical apparatus and a battery of linguistic rules, representations and categories. While I do not suggest that there is anything wrong in this as a heuristic basis for the projection of hypotheses and the generation of research ideas (indeed, it is difficult to see how else research could proceed), it seems to me that this is the least desirable of approaches from the logical point of view. As a consequence, this inevitable research heuristic must not become enshrined as a methodological principle of theory construction, hypothesis confirmation and so on.

Such a 'mixed' strategy may have one of three outcomes. In the first the linguistic categories are reduced to purely psychological categories and the theory becomes a psychological theory of the type already described. In the second the psychological mechanisms become increasingly abstract as they are made to mesh with the linguistic categories until they are indistinguishable from those categories. Such a theory collapses with the linguistic theory type described above. In the third a set of hybrid descriptive and theoretical primes is developed which belong to neither domain. This is inherently undesirable in that it increases the stock of theory types which must be assumed in order to handle the data. This is not to say that such a hybrid theory distinct from psychology or linguistics may never be necessary. However, it is unparsimonious to assume that such a theory will be necessary without exploring all the avenues of inquiry offered by existing theoretical apparatus. Not the least of the problems posed by such hybrids is the difficulty of establishing the ontological interpretive status of the terms of the theory; that is, in deciding precisely what the theory is talking about. Notice that there can be no acceptable fourth outcome. For instance, it will not do to allow a theory which simply mixes categories from psychology and linguistics. This is because the idealisations of linguistic theory detailed in the previous section guarantee that such mixing leads automatically to what philosophers call a category mistake, that is a frank confusion of levels of description.

I shall argue that the only way to conceive of psycholinguistic theory construction is as a development of linguistic theory, and that the logical course of theory construction should therefore involve the deductive strategy. In a later section I shall discuss in detail what appear to me to be attempts to construct a theory of the third type (a mixed theory) and show how such a theory is successful only to the extent that it is reconstrued as a linguistic psycholinguistic theory. I do not believe that the inductive strategy has anything worthwhile to offer psycholinguistics despite the considerable popularity of this mode of reasoning in psychology, artificial intelligence, and amongst some philosophers. However, to establish this point of view even in one limited domain would require far more detailed argument than can be presented here, and would require a more rigorous philosophical discussion than is possible in this chapter. A flavour of the kind of debate I am alluding to can be gained from the pages of Piatelli-Palmarini (1980). See also Atkinson (1982) for critical discussion.

Our aim, then, is to effect a progressive weakening of the idealisations of linguistic theory in such a way as to introduce (still idealised) types of psychological mechanism compatible with the remaining linguistic categories of description. Since idealisations (3) and (6) render linguistic theory literally inapplicable to psycholinguistic theory construction our first task will be to find principled ways to relax these idealisations. The first step will be to introduce a 'stage conception' of learning by relaxing assumption (6) to (6') (cf. White, 1982):

(6') Language acquisition is a function which maps the learner's initial knowledge state, S_0, into a series of states, S_i $(1 < i < n)$. State S_n is the final state (adult knowledge of a particular grammar). In state S_i the learner is ascribed a grammar $G_i \neq G_{i-1}$. Learning is the result of exposure to a degenerate sampling of utterances in the language (not all of them necessarily well-formed) within a perfectly homogeneous speech community.

(6'b) The transition from state S_i to state S_{i+1} $(i < n-1)$ is instantaneous.

I shall refer to each of such states as 'stages'. Notice that nothing in (6') seeks to explain why changes from one stage to another should occur. Furthermore, nothing is said about the length of each stage in real time. The most conservative assumption is that each stage is of negligible duration. Thus, the theory is still a far cry from developmental reality in that the instantaneity assumption is scarcely altered. For interesting discussion of this point see Pinker (1981, 1982). The main difference between such a stage model and the earlier idealisation is that it is now possible to discuss questions concerning the nature of the data the child can use during language learning.

2.2. The mental representation of grammar

In addition to (1)–(6) linguistic theory makes the further assumption (7) (made explicit in e.g. Chomsky, 1965; Chomsky and Halle, 1968):

87

(7) A language user possesses exactly one grammar for all occasions of use and all modalities.

This assumption is regarded by many linguists as being literally true.

Assumption (7) has been questioned in debate concerning the nature of the mental lexicon and access to lexical represent-ations. Butterworth (1983) provides a useful review of the issues. Less cogently, the assumption has been challenged in the context of language disruption in acquired neurological disor-ders. Some have held that an aphasic patient may lose 'compet-ence' in one modality (say, production) while retaining it in another (say, comprehension). (For a review of some of these notions see Lesser, 1978.) Now it is perfectly plain that the facts do not of themselves warrant this conceptual leap, and that other alternatives are if anything more plausible, given the stan-dard construal of the notion of 'competence'. The difficulty lies in distinguishing between the mentally represented grammar and mechanisms for implementing the grammar (cf. also my remarks above on studies on apraxia of speech). At its crudest, discussion of these questions has simply confused psychological levels of description and explanation with linguistic levels. It turns out, then, that relaxing assumption (7) is fraught with conceptual danger. A convincing demonstration of the need to weaken that assumption will be therefore all the more impres-sive.

Suppose we find that it is necessary to describe language processing in different terms for different modalities. There will be one of three explanations available for this:

(i) There is one central grammar and a separate non-linguistic implementation system for each modality.

(ii) For each modality there is a distinct pair consisting of a grammar and its implementation system.

(iii) There is one central general-purpose implementation system and a separate grammar for each modality.

As far as I can tell no-one has ever seriously advanced (iii) so I shall ignore it. From the point of view of linguistic theory the most parsimonious assumption is (i). Adopting this would mean that linguistic theory would have nothing to say about modality differences in language use. However, it would bring with it the prediction that the variability between modalities could be described in non-linguistic terms but could not be described in linguistic terms. If it turned out that the best description of modality differences did appeal to purely linguistic (or at least primarily linguistic) categories, then we would be justified in suspecting that assumption (7) was in need of relaxation. Let us therefore adopt proposal (ii) by relaxing (7) to (7′):

(7′) The language user with n distinct modalities of language use has up to $n + 1$ grammars.

I have made concessions to psychological plausibility in (7′) by suggesting in effect that there might be a distinct grammar for each of the n modalities plus a central grammar which is modality neutral.

The main question posed in this subsection, then, is 'are there any grounds for supposing that there are linguistically definable differences in language processing for any pair of modalities such as would warrant postulation of distinct grammars for those modalities?'. My claim will be that the answer to this question is positive in the domain of articulation development.[3]

3. A THEORY OF ARTICULATION DEVELOPMENT

I have argued in the previous section that psycholinguistic theory construction must proceed by a 'deductive' process in which the idealisations of linguistic theory are successively and systematically relaxed. The development of articulation or 'phonetic competence' (cf. Kiparsky and Menn, 1977) (usually called 'phonological development' rather misleadingly) is a prime example of a psycholinguistic domain that has attracted the attention of linguists, and in which linguistics has had a considerable role to play in theory construction and model building. I shall assume without further comment that this is appropriate, and that therefore a proper theory of articulation development will be constructed out of phonological theory. In this I am joining a tradition which includes Jakobson (1968) and Smith (1973).

Smith's (1973) theory provides a useful starting point for discussion. Smith noted that the machinery of grammatical theory (i.e. the theory of phonology presented in *SPE*) could be put to use to account for the systematic patterning of data found in the speech of his son, Amahl. However, a developing articulation system is very different from the idealised competence of the adult user. In particular, Smith noted that A was able to discriminate far more phonological contrasts than he could reliably distinguish in his own speech at various stages. Furthermore, the *SPE* model of phonology (which, it will be recalled, is in large part a theory of morphophonemics) presupposes abstract underlying representations mapped into surface representations by phonological transformations. This model then provides an account of morphophonemic alternation. However, there is really no obvious equivalent to morphophonemic alternation in early articulation development. Smith therefore reinterpreted the theoretical machinery of *SPE*, not so much relaxing idealisations in the theory, as providing certain formal devices with a very different psychological interpretation. Underlying representations are no longer lexical codings of what is common to alternating allomorphs, but are rather representations of the child's perception of adult *surface* phonological representations. Phonological rules ('realisation rules' in Smith's terminology) are then linguistically defined devices for rendering these perceptual representations pronounceable. (I refer the reader to Smith, 1973, for a more detailed discussion of these points).

Figure 5.1 summarizes Smith's model the technicalities of which are presented in rather more detail in Chapter 6. In that chapter I also present a reanalysis of Smith's work within more contemporary phonological theory, notably autosegmental phonology (cf. also Spencer, 1986). One of the consequences of adopting such an approach is that some of the assumptions of Smith's model are no longer applicable. In particular, an autosegmental account of phenomena such as bidirectional consonant harmony (e.g. 'lateral harmony') demands that a further level of linguistic representation be set up between Smith's level of underlying representation and his level of surface representation. This in turn leads to a bifurcation in the sets of rules linking these levels. It turns out that the intermediate level of representation satisfies linguistic criteria in that it is the point of convergence at which it is possible to define (a) the set of phonemic contrasts the child can articulate; (b) the output of absolute neutralisation processes; (c) underspecification (in a technical sense explained in Chapter 6).

Psychologically interpreted, the extra level of representation induces a distinction between an input store (for the perceptual modality) and an output store (for production). The revised model is shown in Figure 5.2.

Figure 5.1: Smith's (1973) 'classical' model

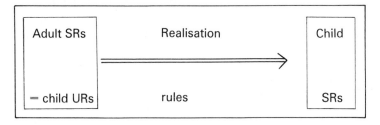

Figure 5.2: Spencer's (1986) revised model (slightly simplified)

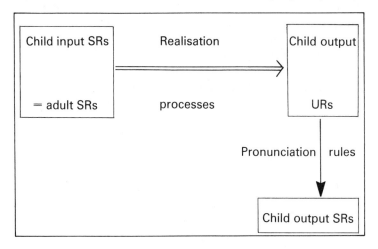

I refer the reader to Spencer (1986) and Chapter 6 (this volume) for further elaboration and justification of the model of Figure 5.2. The points to note are that assumption (7′) (with $n=2$) is implicit in this model, and that the weakening of assumption (7) this entails has been motivated solely by linguistic reasoning. In the light of discussion at the end of the previous section it is also worth remarking that the model presupposes linguistically defined processes linking modality-specific sets of stored representations (lexicons) but that it in no way presupposes that a representation of those processes is involved in on-line language use or in development. Finally, it ought to be stressed that the model is actually only minimally different from the classical model of Smith (1973), when recent advances in phonological theory are taken into consideration. In particular, no component of the model is motivated solely by non-linguistic psychological principles. This means that there is very little danger of the confusion of levels of description against which I have been regularly warning.

3.2. Menn's theory

Proposals with roughly the content of Figure 5.2 have been advanced before in the literature, e.g. by Ingram (1974, 1976), Menn, and others. Perhaps the most articulated theory of this sort, and the one that is most readily comparable with the theory developed here, is that of Menn (1979), whose model is illustrated in Figure 5.3 (certain details of Menn's model, which have been suppressed here for expositional reasons, are briefly discussed in Spencer, 1986).

Figure 5.3: Menn's (1979) model (simplified)

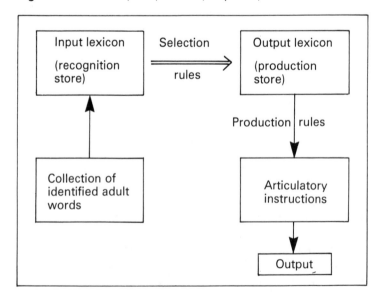

The 'production rules' in Figure 5.3 seem to correspond roughly to what I have labelled 'pronunciation rules' in Figure 5.2. The output lexicon is a set of stored representations subserving just pronunciation, a level or representation distinct from that of the input lexicon which subserves just perception. Menn's 'selection rules' have presumably roughly the same function as my 'realisation processes', in that they effect a mapping from input to output stores. However, it is not clear from Menn's discussion how any of these levels of representation or sets of processes is to be characterised or individuated. For instance, she does not adopt an autosegmental model of phonological analysis (though see her programmatic suggestions in Menn, 1978), and, of course, her model largely predates theories appealing to underspecification. Yet these linguistic formalisms play an important role in determining the structure of the model in Figure 5.2. Thus, despite the topological similarity between Figures 5.2 and 5.3 it is not immediately apparent how Menn's model relates to mine.[4]

Figure 5.3 does not include one piece of theoretical apparatus used by Menn: the output constraint. An output constraint is a statement to the effect that certain sounds or combinations of sounds are not permitted. It thus largely corresponds with what linguists call a phonotactic constraint. The output constraint is included by Menn to provide motivation for the operation of phonological rules (such as   final consonant devoicing) by stating directly the phonotactic constraint embodied in the rule.

Smith (1978) has criticised this conception on the grounds that it includes theoretical apparatus which is not warranted. Unfortunately, given the state of play at the time Smith was writing, there was very little evidence that machinery over and above that of the classical model of Smith (1973) was needed. (The only alteration Smith introduced was a perceptual filter to account for occasional mishearings; this was prompted by the linguistic reanalysis of his data provided by Macken, 1980.) Smith showed that given current assumptions the input/output distinction was otiose, and that this was particularly true of the output constraints.

The output constraints are not phonological well-formedness conditions or phonotactic constraints of the usual kind, otherwise there would be no need to include them along with the phonological rules (cf. Smith, 1978). On the other hand their purpose is to 'restrict and motivate' phonological rules. Now, if they are not defined at the phonological level of description they must presumably be defined at a psycholinguistic level of processing. But then they cannot interact with rules as such, only with psycholinguistic processes corresponding descriptively to the linguistic rules. But in that case the rules Menn speaks of are not phonological rules, but rather they are psycholinguistic processes. Yet they are presented as phonological rules and have the format of phonological rules. As far as I can tell Menn would not subscribe to the view that articulation development has to be described in purely psychological, non-linguistic terms, at least not at the present state of research.

In attempting to make sense of Menn's output constraints we thus find ourselves going round in circles. This is symptomatic of a classical confusion of levels of description. Menn's position can, however, be salvaged, along with most of the details of her model, if we take as our starting point a linguistic description of the phenomena to be addressed. In that case either we formalise the data in terms of phonological rules, or in terms of output constraints, or we may formalise some processes in terms of the one device and other processes in terms of the other. What we do not do, if we are to adhere to linguistic methodology, is set up two distinct explanations for the same set of facts. I have chosen to code some of the facts in terms of rules (more properly universal conditions on association and so on) and other facts in terms of well-formedness conditions on underlying representations in the output lexicon (see Chapter 6 this volume). In this way our theory remains consistent, and we avoid the trap of mixing linguistic and psycholinguistic levels of description.

This illustrates a not uncommon phenomenon of a theory being more or less correct, but for the wrong reasons. The suspicion, based on intuitions about the psycholinguistics of development, that input and output stores were distinct, could not be demonstrated given the assumptions of classical generative phonology (assumptions which Menn largely shared at that point). Ironically, Smith's model was preferable until a more powerful and revealing variety of phonological theory became available.[5]

4. INTERIM SUMMARY CONCLUSIONS

I have argued that the historical tendency in developmental phonological studies towards taking a variety of linguistic theory and applying it to child language data should be promoted to a methodological principle. Proceeding from a presentation of the standard ideality assumptions of theoretical linguistics (generative grammar) I showed how a psycholinguistic theory could be constructed by a process of systematically relaxing those idealisations. Furthermore, I have claimed that only this strategy will provide a coherent psycholinguistic *theory*, as opposed to isolated models of local aspects of development or mere descriptions of the facts.

Choice of recent so-called 'non-linear' theories of phonology demands a model of development which includes separate levels of representation on the input and output sides. The resulting model is justified solely by linguistic analysis, without recourse to speculation about psycholinguistic processing. The model was compared with Menn's almost identical model, which avowedly takes as its starting point presumed psycholinguistic mechanisms and constraints. I showed that there were difficulties in interpreting that model, however. Moreover, I pointed out that given the model of phonology which Menn was presupposing there was no reason why she should need to postulate a model more articulated than the 'classical' model, unless she were to adopt a purely psychological model and abandon the view that phonological analysis had any role to play in modelling articulation development.

The resulting model is maximally parsimonious in that it appeals to the minimum of theoretical baggage and makes fewest assumptions. As a consequence it is still a highly idealised theory. (For instance, on this theory language learning still takes place instantaneously.) This means that there are a great many experimentally or observationally established facts of phonological development that cannot be incorporated into the theory. For instance, frequently reported observations such as selective avoidance, favourite sounds, the 'fis' phenomenon and so on (for a textbook review see Edwards and Shriberg, 1983) remain outside the purview of the theory. This is no shortcoming, however. For there is no rival theory into which such facts can be incorporated. Furthermore, given our present understanding it is hard to see how a coherent theory could be

95

proposed which would be able to accommodate such findings in a principled manner.

The theory enshrined in Figure 5.2 leaves a good many questions unanswered. Some of the more important ones are:

(i) How is 'real' phonology learnt?

(ii) What is the relationship between phonological development and the development of other aspects of language (notably syntax and morphology)?

(iii) How is suprasegmental phonology developed and how does it relate to segmental phonological development?

(iv) How does phonological development relate to the development of auditory/perceptual skills and phonetic motor skills?

(v) How does the developmental theory relate to models of childhood performance including slips of the tongue, learning strategies (see above), etc?

(vi) How does the theory relate to questions of abnormal development (especially speech and language pathology such as phonological disability)?

(vii) What are the implications of the developmental theory for theories of adult phonology, speech perception/production etc? In particular, is the input/output distinction required for understanding adult language use?

I leave these as questions for future research. I turn now to a consideration of recent discussion of psycholinguistic theory construction in the domain of developmental psycholinguistics in an attempt to put my observations into a broader philosophical setting.

5. CRITERIA OF EXPLANATORY ADEQUACY

A detailed and penetrating critique has been provided of developmental psycholinguistic theorising by Atkinson (1982). Atkinson couches his discussion in the context of the philosophy of science, and asks whether theories of child language development (or language acquisition) meet a series of conditions of adequacy which, claims Atkinson, any theory of development ought ideally meet. In this section I measure the theory of phonological development discussed here against Atkinson's conditions. For reasons of space I shall not weigh other theories against these conditions, though it should be obvious that I regard my proposals as matching up to Atkinson's criteria rather better than other theories.

It should be pointed out that Atkinson is sceptical of competence theories ('the axiomatisation of a range of possibilities') presented as psychological theories, preferring what he refers to as the 'traditional position', in which 'psychological explanations have involved the formulation of laws relating mental states and observable behaviour' (1982, p. 6). I briefly take up this point later. Nonetheless, Atkinson points out that most acquisition theories 'have to be construed as competence theories if they are to be intelligible' and that 'this mode of psychological theorising has not, as yet, received the critical attention which it undoubtedly deserves' (1982, p. 7). One might add that this mode of theorising has not received much in the way of *sympathetic* attention, either.

Atkinson formulates five conditions of adequacy on purportedly explanatory theories in developmental psycholinguistics. They are reproduced below (taken from Atkinson's own summary (1982, p. 25)). In these conditions T is construed as a sequence $(T_1, \ldots, T_n, M)$ where $T_1, \ldots, T_n$ is a sequence of theories designed to explain the behaviour of the child at various stages of development, and M is a learning mechanism. All five conditions are predicated over a theory T in the domain D of language development.

CONDITION I

T is an explanatory theory in D only if T_i is an explanatory theory in D at T_i $(1 \leqslant i \leqslant n)$, where the predicate 'is an explanatory theory in D at t' relies for its explication on adopting some view on the general problem of explanation in psychology.

CONDITION II

T is (standardly) an explanatory theory in D only if T_i is constructed in accordance with a particular general theory $(1 \leqslant i \leqslant n)$. This ensures that the T_i are comparable in the required sense. If the T_i are not so constructed then additional argument may restore the explanatory status of T.

CONDITION IIIa

If T admits of analysis in terms of additive complexity, then T is

97

an explanatory theory in D only if T_{i+1} is additively more complex than T_i $(1 \leqslant i \leqslant n)$.

CONDITION IIIb
Where D is a domain of constraints, if T admits of analysis in terms of additive complexity, then T is an explanatory theory in D only if T_{i+1} is less complex than T_i $(1 \leqslant i \leqslant n)$.

CONDITION IV
T is an explanatory theory in D only if the sequence of theories $(T_1, \ldots, T_n)$ admits of a teleological, a reductive or an environmental explanation.

CONDITION V
T is an explanatory theory in D only if M is specified in such a way as to explain the transition from T_i to T_{i+1} on the basis of data available at t_{i+1} $(1 \leqslant i \leqslant n)$.

The intuitive content of Condition I is that acquisition theory must be grounded. Atkinson presents this as uncontroversial. Condition II serves to guarantee that there will be no conceptual discontinuities between different theoretical stages of development. Conditions III demand that the development theories characterising each stage should get more complex as development itself increases in complexity. (Atkinson is deliberately vague as to what he means by complexity here.) Condition IV demands that some explanation be forthcoming as to why change takes place in the way it does. Condition V is simply a demand for a theory of learnability.

The theory proposed here is grounded in the theory of generative grammar, and it presupposes the ontological commitments of that theory. It is not clear that Atkinson would admit this as adequate, but nor is it clear what Atkinson would regard as adequate grounding, at least in the domain of articulation development. I discuss this further below.

Condition II says that the subtheories proposed for each developmental stage should be globally comparable. This is satisfied (near-)trivially. The principled method of theory construction by which idealistions are systematically relaxed covers all stages of development. The only possible problem that I can envisage concerns the fate of the separation between input and output lexicons. I have remained agnostic about how the final state is characterised with respect to this distinction (cf.

question (vii) section 5). However, there is no reason to believe that the theory will commit us to any discontinuity here.

I am unsure how much my theory adheres to Condition III. I follow Smith (1973) in assuming that the child starts out with a set of rules (realisation processes and pronunciation rules in my case) which he loses as his articulation improves. On the face of it, it appears then that I am characterising development as the diminution of complexity, rather than the reverse. I see no alternative, however. Well-known phenomena such as phonological idioms, 'recidivism' and the like show that children do not misarticulate because they are physically unable to articulate, but rather because they find it advantageous to impose simplifications on phonological representations. These can be likened to the compensatory strategies observed in any other form of motor skill acquisition. In this respect my theory is no different from Smith's and both, I believe, are perfectly well motivated. (Recall that Atkinson simply does not discuss any aspects of language development that are best regarded as skill acquisition rather than the acquisition of underlying competence.)

However, I believe there is one way in which my theory is an improvement over Smith's with regard to Condition III. In Smith's theory the only level of representation at which complexity increases with development is the level of the child's surface forms. This is the minimum concession which can be made to Condition III. In the present theory, however, there is an extra level of representation, corresponding to the knowledge which underlies the child's articulatory skill. The representations at this level (that of the output lexicon) increase in complexity as the child is able to make more contrasts. Thus, there is a level of representation in the theory which conforms very well to Condition III.

Condition IV demands that developmental theory provide some sort of rationale for the sequence of development observed. Atkinson provides three alternative types of rationale: teleological, reductive and environmental.

The teleological rationale is akin to the 'intrinsic ordering' of rules in a grammar. If a stage of development has to precede some other stage because it furnishes the logical prerequisites for the appearance of the later stage then the ordering is explained teleologically. For instance, to use an example Atkinson himself cites, if a theory posits the acquisition of transformational syntactic rules and phrase structure rules, then some at least of the latter have to be acquired before any of the former, by virtue of the formal nature of the rules themselves. This provides strong justification for the ordering of stages.

A reductive explanation accounts for the developmental sequence in terms of some other, more basic or general, theory of psychology or physiology or whatever. In our case such an explanation would appeal to articulatory or perceptual phonetics or to general cognitive principles. From what little is known about the physiology and psychophysics of articulation development it seems unlikely that principled reduction to these domains will be feasible. The chances of general cognitive principles offering any explanatory account seem even more remote in the case of articulation development than in the case of other areas of language development.

If we explain developmental sequences in terms of the order in which relevant data are presented to the child (by the environment, as it were) then we have the third, environmental, type of explanation. Now, there is much that needs to be learnt regarding the data children have available about the sound pattern of their language. This is of greatest relevance to theories of phonological perception, however, an aspect of development I have ignored for expositional reasons. A number of baroque possibilities come to mind, interpretable as environmental explanations for articulation development, but they do not seem worth pursuing at the present stage of research.

To the extent that the theory meets Condition IV, then, it does so by virtue of 'teleology'. While the kinds of teleological explanations Atkinson has in mind don't carry over automatically (for reasons to be discussed) nevertheless, it seems that some of the explanatory value of the present theory flows from its formal properties in the desired way. The crucial components of the theory are that there is an input lexicon and an output lexicon linked by neutralising realisation processes, and the output lexicon is mapped onto the child's actual output by a set of 'pronunciation rules' defined phonologically. Further, the number of contrasts represented in the input lexicon is never less than the number represented on the output side.

Part of articulation development is coded as the loss of the filter between input and output lexicons. To some extent, then, the course of development is a consequence of our assumption that the output lexicon represents no more contrasts than the input lexicon. At the same time the 'pronunciation rules', which account for the equivalent of allophonic variation on the output side, change and are ultimately lost as development proceeds. It turns out that some of these rules (notably autosegmental processes) are dependent for their form on the structure of the output lexical entries. The example discussed in some detail in Spencer (1986, Chapter 6 this volume) in which a process of 'labial attraction' is lost simultaneously with a process of cluster reduction is of this type. Thus, while in general there is no teleological reason for the course of development, such an explanation is forthcoming for certain individual processes, again by virtue of the formal properties of the linguistic theory underlying the psycholinguistic model. Indeed, I present this particular case as one of the stronger arguments in favour of my theory over Smith's original. The conclusion is that teleological explanations for interesting subparts of the theory are forthcoming. I believe this is one of the more important areas in which my theory enjoys advantages over others.

The conditions on Atkinson's list which are problematical in the present context are Conditions I and V. The reasons for this are interesting. Condition V is in essence a call for a theory of learnability. Not surprisingly he presents the work of Wexler and Culicover (1980) as a paradigm of this approach (though nowadays one ought include the discursive learning theory of Pinker, 1984). These authors devote little more than a paragraph to the problem of learnability theory for 'real' phonology, and don't address the question of articulation development at all.[6]

Although Atkinson opens his discussion of developmental psycholinguistics with a detailed account of Jakobson's (1968) theory of phonological development, he largely ignores other work in the field of developmental phonology in the rest of the book. His only reference to learnability is the observation that Jakobson does not provide an explicit learning mechanism. Unfortunately, comparison of generative theories of phonological development with Jakobson's Praguian theory is misleading. Jakobson did not make the now common assumption that children internalise the adult surface phonemic system (more or less) at an early stage. Therefore, it is perfectly possible to recast Jakobson's research as a theory of the development of something like a 'classical' competence. As Atkinson points out, there are serious difficulties of interpretation here, largely because Jakobson concentrates on production data to the exclusion of perceptual data, but at least his theory has roughly the same shape as the other theories of grammatical development Atkinson discusses. Generative theories, however, such as the present one, have an entirely different character.

A generative theory of phonological development (including Stampean natural phonology) in effect sidesteps the important learnability question entirely, by assuming that the child has already acquired the adult surface system. The primary research question (as should be very evident from the present model) is then 'what mental transformations are performed over phonological representations during that process of motor skill acquisition which constitutes the development of articulation?'. It is by no means clear what constitutes a learnability problem here. In a sense the child has 'learnt' everything he needs to know inasmuch as he has some representation at least of the adult surface forms he is trying to articulate.

This problem is highlighted in the present theory (given assumption 7′) which allows us to modularise linguistic knowledge. For it is now no longer clear what learning consists of. Suppose that we attribute to one modality a set of representations, rules or whatever, lacking in another modality, and that development is construed as the development of those rules and representations in the second modality interacting with the first. In this case the learnability problem will assume different proportions. For if one modality has already acquired the relevant linguistic knowledge then the learnability problem is trivially solved. On the other hand, the acquisition of that knowledge by the second modality is perhaps better seen as a species of cross-modal integration rather than as learning proper.

Assuming that these questions can be given adequate clarification, I would claim that my theory both fails and succeeds on Atkinson's fifth condition. It fails in the sense that it presupposes a largely correct parsing of incoming phonological representations from a very early stage, but makes no attempt to explain how this is achieved (any more than most other theorists do). It succeeds in that it provides a restrictive basis for projecting hypotheses about the correct pronunciation of a word, namely the phonological component of UG (in particular, syllable structure constraints, procedures for effecting underspecification of lexical entries and so on). Implicit in the model is the assumption that only universally allowable rules/representation systems are available to the child. This is an inherent property of the theory as it has been developed. Admittedly, success in this respect is not as spectacular as that achieved in natural phonology (Stampe, 1979). In Stampe's theory, phonological processes are innate and are suppressed as development proceeds. A close and ingenious link is thus forged between development and adult phonological systems. Unfortunately, there is evidence that Stampe's proposals are too strong (see below, section 6). The nearest equivalent to Stampe's strong nativism in the generative phonology presupposed here is a somewhat inexplicit theory of markedness.

Failure to provide a learning mechanism of the depth and sophistication of that of recent work in learnability theory is not too damning. Much of the indeterminacy can be traced to ignorance about universals of phonology. Where the present theory outstrips its competitors is in the close connection between the developmental theory and phonological theory: gains made in the latter can readily be incorporated into the former, provided the psycholinguistic theory cleaves to linguistic theory in the manner I have advocated. If the psycholinguistic theory has any source other than linguistic theory it is hardly likely that a sensible attack will be made on Condition V.

What merits particular attention from this discussion is that even the more articulated theories of articulation development have next to nothing to say about *learning*. The problem of how children acquire their input representations has been uniformly ignored (but see Waterson, 1971; Chiat, 1979). This is worrying for two main reasons — one theoretical, one practical.

The theoretical problem concerns the nature of the adult surface representations which by common consent provide the data for learning. Central to the present theory is the notion of lexical contrast. Conventional generative wisdom has had it that the notion of surface phonemic contrast is derivative, and that the only notion of interest to phonological theory is that of underlying contrast. Ideas reminiscent of structuralist phonemics have made a reappearance in the recent generative literature (e.g. Mohanan's (1982) notion of lexical representation. See also Kiparsky (1985) for extremely interesting discussion of these trends.), but a theory which relies on children in effect having a discovery procedure for taxonomic phonemics defined over surface representations owes current linguistic theory something of an explanation.

The practical problem concerns the role of misperception or misstorage in disorders of articulation (so-called 'phonological disorders'). It seems very likely that inaccurate coding accounts for an important subpopulation of children presenting clinically with disordered speech but lacking overt pathology (see Dinnsen, Elbert and Weismer, 1981; Spencer, Chapter 6 this volume). Current models of analysis and assessment based on phonological theory hardly take any account of this aspect of learning. Without a theory of how such storage is achieved by normal children it is difficult to see how much progress can be made in this very important area of speech pathology.

Returning to Atkinson's Condition I, it should be obvious that we are dealing here with the cognitive determinants of motor skill acquisition and not with the acquisition of knowledge of grammar. But if we pursue this line of argument then all discussion of Atkinson's conditions of adequacy on explanatory theories of language development appears to be beside the point. For on this view learning to talk is more like learning to ride a bicycle or learning to play the piano. But if this is the case why do we take linguistic theory as our point of departure in constructing a theory of articulation development?

The simple answer to this last question is that the data pattern in a linguistic fashion. Attempts to apply linguistic techniques of analysis to child production data have met with enormous success; much more so than in other areas of language development, and this despite the fact that in general by no means the full power of phonological theory has been turned onto the problem. It is simply inconceivable that this is coincidental. The obvious conclusion is that the motor skill concerned is governed by a rich cognitive system which at a certain level of description receives its best characterisation in linguistic theory. A similar viewpoint has been urged in the domain of adult speech production theory (see Hammarberg, 1976, 1982). Presumably it is speech production theory, and more generally the theory of motor skills, which is supposed to provide the grounding of a developmental theory of articulation, if we take Condition I seriously. Unfortunately, motor skills theory in general is poorly developed. The area is highly controversial precisely because of serious dissent over how much emphasis to place on cognitive, representational determinants of behaviour. While some (Schmidt, 1976; Stelmach, 1978) place reliance on mentally represented 'motor programs' governing performance, others, working within the paradigm of 'ecological psychology' championed by J. Gibson (Turvey, 1977, and many other references within so-called Action Theory), vigorously deny the coherence of appealing to a representational theory. (For application of this mode of reasoning to speech production see Fowler, Rubin, Remez and Turvey, 1980; for a highly readable textbook presentation of the debates see Kelso, 1982.)

The outcome of these extremely interesting developments is irrelevant to my present argument. The point is that there is no agreed theory of speech production which could ground a developmental theory of articulation in accordance with Condition I. More seriously, if we were to try to interpret a linguistically based psycholinguistic theory in terms of 'some view on the general problem of explanation in psychology' we would be immediately confronted with a difficult choice: whether to opt for a non-representational (neo-Gibsonian, 'ecological') theory or a representational, cognitive theory. We would then find that if we opted for the latter at least one influential set of models of speech production was related to linguistic theory in precisely the same way that the generative theory of articulation development is related to linguistic theory. For according to this view a non-linguistic theory of phonetics (and hence of speech production) is incoherent (cf. Hammarberg, 1982). I conclude from this that in the domain of developmental phonology Condition I is far from straightforward, and, in fact, to insist upon it betokens a simplistic attitude to the problem of explanation in psychology.

To conclude this evaluation, when we recognise that the theory is essentially a theory of the cognitive determinants of motor skill acquisition and not a theory of grammar learning proper, the theory fares very well against Atkinson's stringent metatheoretical injunctions, at least in respect of those conditions which can be accepted as relatively uncontroversial in our domain. While I have not been able to prove this assertion, it is my belief that this success is a direct consequence of the stance taken on psycholinguistic theory construction, namely that the psycholinguistic theory should be derived from linguistic theory by means of minimal relaxation of ideality assumptions. Nor is this a consequence of bias within Atkinson's conditions. As I have suggested, Atkinson himself would appear to be sceptical of the role of linguistic metatheoretical assumptions in psychology.

6. CLINICAL PHONOLOGY

Much of my discussion has been technical if not philosophical. It might be thought that this was very far removed from the practical concerns of clinical researchers or practitioners. Unfortunately, this is not the case. Almost any foray into the nature of human cognition will bring the investigator face to face with epistemological questions of some complexity. Insensitivity to this has led to confusion in the past and, left uncorrected, cannot but hinder research. A good example of this in the area of acquired neurological disorders is charted by Buckingham (1980) in his discussion of the confusions surrounding the nature of apraxia of speech. Buckingham points out that a laxness in the application of linguistic concepts such as 'phoneme' has led to serious conceptual confusion in the apraxia literature. Much of the debate over whether apraxia of speech is a motor disorder or a linguistic disorder is incoherent by virtue of this confusion. The questions I have been raising are thus of more than academic interest. For patients, the penalty of confusion on the part of clinicians can be severe if entire treatment programmes are built upon false premises.

Research into phonological development is unusual in that a very high proportion of recent research findings have been gleaned from clinical populations rather than normally developing children. This is partly due to the importance of therapy in this area, and partly due to the interest that has been excited by the possibility of applying techniques of phonological analysis to clinical problems.

In many cases, unfortunately, research has been marred by a failure to understand the linguistic methodology or principles which are being applied. Parker (1976) discusses the way distinctive feature theory has been misapplied in clinical contexts, and Carney (1979) is rightly critical of attempts to develop an assessment tool based solely on a distinctive feature analysis of children's productions (McReynolds and Engmann, 1975). Attempts to apply markedness theory to clinical problems have been made (e.g. Marquardt, Reinhart and Peterson, 1979) but it seems to me that this is putting the cart before the horse. At the present very crude state of understanding of markedness, it makes more sense to let the facts of speech disorders determine the nature of markedness theory rather than the other way round. I think too much could be made of the inadequacies of these attempts, however. I would contend that the real problem that clinical researchers face is not so much their own impoverished understanding of linguistics (though misunderstanding of linguistic theory is always something to be on guard against) but rather the lack of a clearly articulated psycholinguistic theory of development that researchers can work within.

By far the most influential trend in clinical phonology in recent years has been so-called phonological process analysis (PPA), developed originally by David Ingram (1976; see also Ingram, 1981; Weiner, 1979, 1984. A good textbook review of PPA and its progenitor, Natural Phonology, is provided in Edwards and Shriberg, 1983). I confess that in many respects I find the current emphasis on PPA somewhat disquieting. There are two reasons for this. First, I do not believe that the linguistic theory underlying PPA has a great deal to offer psycholinguistic theory construction. Second, even if that theory did provide a suitable basis for a theory of articulation development, the way that PPA tends to be applied suggests that its purpose and nature has been widely misconstrued. To the extent that this criticism is valid it is because users of PPA have tended to regard it as a linguistic technique to be applied directly to clinical data without the intervention of an appropriate theory of language use, particularly, articulation development. I discuss each of these difficulties in turn.

Phonological Process Analysis is derived historically from the theory of Natural Phonology propounded by Stampe some 15 years ago (see Stampe, 1979; Donegan and Stampe, 1979). In this theory Stampe postulates an intimate connection between the nature of phonological theory and the nature of a theory of phonological (more properly, articulation) development. He assumes that the child has available a perfect perceptual command of the adult surface system of phonemic contrasts (cf. Smith) and that his own articulation is the result of applying 'phonological processes', a variety of phonological rule motivated by phonetic 'naturalness', to those representations. These processes are provided innately and can be extrinsically ordered, and the child has no choice at the outset but to apply them. However, by altering the format of the processes, or by suppressing them altogether or by reordering them, the child gradually brings his pronunciation into line with the adult system. Some of the processes are never lost or modified, and

107

these become part of the systematic phonology of the adult language.

The view that the processes children apply to derive their output forms must be 'natural' has been challenged (Kiparsky and Menn, 1977). Even beyond the early 'first 50-word' stage, children seem to experiment with phonological processes (or rules) which should not be countenanced in Stampe's theory. Another problem is that for Stampe, all the processes found in normally developing speech should correspond to some sort of natural phonological process in a fully fledged adult system. Yet there are very common phenomena in child language which have little or no reflex in adult phonologies. For example, although varieties of consonant harmony are reported in a number of languages these generally involve nasals or sibilants (e.g. a number of languages of America and Africa only allow a [s] or a [ʃ] in a word but not both). Conspicuously absent, however, are assimilation of velars to dentals ('fronting'), or vice-versa ('backing') or a phenomenon almost universal amongst learners of English, 'lateral harmony', by which median approximants are assimilated to [l]. While it is not uncommon to find allophonic variation between varieties of /l/ and median approximants I know of no case of a *harmony* rule of this kind. Admittedly, many of the processes found in children's speech do seem to correspond to adult phonological rules, and it is possible that this is connected with the way articulation develops, but it would appear that Stampe's own strongly nativist explanation of this observation needs to be tempered considerably. Finally, and for me very persuasively, it seems very difficult to maintain Stampe's essentially 'classical' model of articulation development and employ the linguistic techniques of non-linear analysis and underspecification. Put differently, natural phonology does not seem to provide the best account of phonology and so *a fortiori* it cannot provide the best account of developing phonology.

When we look at the way PPA is used clinically it is clear that certain aspects of Stampe's theory have been taken over without modification to the clinical domain. For instance, it is almost universally assumed in the clinical literature that the child's underlying form is identical to the adult surface form, otherwise the whole process of PPA couldn't get off the ground. It is unlikely that Stampe would make such an assumption himself for clinical data, but judging from the almost total lack of discussion of the problem it appears as though the question has not even occurred to many PPA users. Yet as Dinnsen and his colleagues have pointed out (Dinnsen *et al.*, 1981) not only is this a dubious assumption, but if standard techniques of phonological analysis are employed — in particular, if regular alternations and intra-lexical free variation are used to establish underlying forms — it turns out that some children appear to have underlying contrasts which are neutralised (or at least altered; cf. Dinnsen, 1985) while others simply do not have the underlying contrast in the first place.

In keeping with Stampe's theory it is generally assumed that articulation development is characterised by the suppression of processes. In addition, processes may be altered so as to apply to a different set of inputs. However, it is extremely rare for analyses to be presented in the clinical literature of development characterised in terms of the re-ordering of processes. It is perhaps unsurprising that this aspect of Stampe's theory should have been underplayed given the difficulty of providing analyses that take ordering into account, and the conceptual problem of making psycholinguistic or clinical sense of the idea of re-ordering a pair of processes. Nonetheless, this omission makes it more difficult to relate clinical analytic practice to the underlying theory.

Part of the reason for these difficulties stems from an ambivalence towards Stampe's theory on the part of the pioneers of the PPA approach, especially Ingram. Ingram (1976, pp. 4, 48ff.) explicitly states that he rejects Stampe's views on the accuracy of perception even in normal development, and offers a compromise between Stampe's position and that of Jakobson based on Piagetian developmental theory. Not unnaturally, given the state of the art at that time, Ingram is unable to provide a very deep or coherent theory of the relationship between perception and production, and as far as I can see the Piagetian emphasis is a red herring (though his ideas on the interplay between perception and production are very interesting and deserve closer scrutiny). But if the arguments of this chapter are valid Ingram has cut himself off from the conceptual underpinnings he needs for a theory of abnormal phonological development by rejecting Stampe's basis while retaining his techniques of analysis. There has, of course, been much interesting programmatic work concerned with these questions. Waterson (1971 and 1987) presents a perceptually biased theory of development, but this is of little help to Ingram, for it is constructed, in effect, by relaxing ideality assumptions of a very different type of phonological theory, prosodic phonology (not that Waterson would regard her theory in these terms, of course). Furthermore, a great many interesting proposals have been forthcoming from Ferguson and his colleagues in Stanford; but no really satisfactory theoretical basis has been found to fill the vacuum.

I offer these criticisms in a constructive spirit. None of them vitiates the use of PPA as a clinical tool, or even as a research tool. My point is simply that a great deal of painstaking work has to be done at the level of theory construction before this approach can be regarded as an alternative to a theory constructed in the way I have been advocating. Moreover, it is my suspicion that attempts to place such work on a firmer theoretical footing will ultimately end up producing a psycholinguistic theory which is related to linguistic theory in precisely the way I say it must be.

NOTES

1. There is a minor wrinkle here. A good deal is made of so-called 'poverty of stimulus' arguments in theoretical linguistics, according to which a structural property of UG is advanced on the grounds that it could not be inductively discerned by the learner from the data he has available. However, it is not clear how this 'degeneracy of data' assumption interacts with the 'instantaneity of acquisition' assumption, since if a language is learned instantaneously then the type of data in principle available to the learner is indeterminate. I shall assume that this is merely a technical problem of no substantive interest.

2. This means that the notion 'competence theory' is relative. For example, an intermediate theory will be a 'performance theory' relative to a pure competence theory, and a 'competence theory' relative to a pure performance theory.

3. Stabler (1983) has argued that there is no obvious way in which the grammars proposed by linguists could be incorporated into a computational psychological theory as represented systems, presupposing what he calls a third-level theory. In other words there is no evidence that language use involves computations over a *representation* of the grammar. This is to be distinguished from his second-level theory in which language use involves computations over mental representations and those computations and representations can most appropriately be described in linguistic terms, but in which there is no sense in which a superordinate representation of the linguist's grammar governs the computations themselves.

One of the reasons why multiple grammars are unattractive to linguists is that if a representation of the grammar governs language use it makes no sense to have more than one such representation. However, if a mentally represented grammar is not involved the way is open for separate modalities to have their own specially compiled version of the grammar, tailor-made in a 'domain-specific' way for separate 'modules' (cf. Fodor, 1983) of language use such as input and output systems. On the other hand, if there are good reasons for accepting domain-specific systems behaving like modified grammars, this strengthens Stabler's arguments against the existence of a single mentally represented grammar.

4. This in itself is a cautionary tale. At the superficial and crude level of analysis represented by 'box and arrows' models very few conclusions can be drawn about the relationships between different theoretical accounts of the same domain. What is needed is as accurate a characterisation as possible of each of the theoretical constructs in such a model. One of the corollaries of this chapter is that in psycholinguistic research it is linguistic theory which offers the most powerful tools for providing such a characterisation.

5. A personal anecdote is instructive here. My early attempts at reanalysis of Smith (1973) were shelved in 1983, because I found myself needing to postulate what I thought was an unwarranted type of underlying zero specification, with blank-filling redundancy rules intermingling with feature-specifying phonological rules. With the advent of Archangeli's (1984) thesis it became apparent that such a form of grammatical organisation could be justified after all, and the rest of the reanalysis slotted neatly into place.

6. Isolated programmatic remarks on the learnability problem in 'real' phonology are found in the literature (e.g. McCarthy, 1981; Dresher, 1981) but I have seen no systematic account (but cf. Dresher and Kaye, 1986, for interesting discussion).

REFERENCES

Archangeli, D. (1984) *Underspecification in Yawelmani phonology and morphology*, MIT, PhD dissertation

Atkinson, M. (1982) *Explanation in the study of language development*, Cambridge University Press, Cambridge

Buckingham, H. (1980) Explanations of the concept of apraxia of speech. In M. Sarno (ed.), *Acquired aphasia*, Academic Press, London

Butterworth, B. (1983) Lexical representation. In B. Butterworth, (ed.), *Language production*, vol. 2, Academic Press, London

Carney, E. (1979) Inappropriate abstraction in speech-assessment procedures. *British Journal of Disorders of Communication, 14*, 123-35

Chiat, S. (1979) The role of the word in phonological development. *Linguistics, 17*, 591-610

Chomsky, N. (1965) *Aspects of the theory of syntax*, MIT Press,

Cambridge, Mass.

Chomsky, N. (1975) *Reflections on language*, Fontana, London

Chomsky, N. (1980) *Rules and representations*, Blackwell, Oxford

Chomsky, N. (1981) *Lectures on government and binding*, Foris, Dordrecht

Chomsky, N. and Halle, M. (1968) *The sound pattern of English*, Harper & Row, New York

Dinnsen, D. (1985) A re-examination of phonological neutralization. *Journal of Linguistics, 21*, 265-80

Dinnsen, D., Elbert, M. and Weismer, G. (1981) Some typological properties of functional misarticulating systems. In W.O. Dressler (ed.), *Phonologica 1980*, Innsbrucker Beitrage zur Sprachwissenschaft, Innsbruck

Donegan, P. and Stampe, D. (1979) The study of Natural Phonology. In D. Dinnsen (ed.), *Current approaches to phonological theory*, Indiana University Press, Bloomington

Dresher, B.E. (1981) On the learnability of abstract phonology. In C. Baker and J. McCarthy (eds), *The logical problem of language acquisition*, MIT Press, Cambridge, Mass.

Dresher, B.E. and Kaye, J. (1986) Talk delivered at GLOW Colloquium Workshop, Girona

Edwards, M.-L. and Shriberg, L. (1983) *Phonology*, College-Hill Press, Baltimore

Ferguson, C. and Farwell, C. (1975) Words and sounds in early language acquisition. *Language, 51* 419-39.

Fodor, J.A. (1983) *Modularity of mind*, MIT Press, Cambridge, Mass.

Fowler, C., Rubin, A., Remez, R. and Turvey, M. (1980) Implications for speech production of a general theory of action. In B. Butterworth (ed.), *Language production*, vol. 1, Academic Press, London

Frazier, L. and Fodor, J.D. (1978) The sausage machine: a new two-stage parsing model. *Cognition, 6*, 291-325

Hammarberg, R. (1976) The metaphysics of coarticulation. *Journal of Phonetics, 4* 353-63

Hammarberg, R. (1982) On redefining coarticulation. *Journal of Phonetics, 10*, 123-37

Ingram, D. (1974) Phonological rules in young children. *Journal of Child Language, 1*, 49-64.

Ingram, D. (1976) *Phonological disability in children*, Arnold, London

Ingram, D. (1981) *Procedures for the phonological analysis of children's language*, University Park Press, Baltimore

Jakobson, R. (1968) *Child language, aphasia and phonological universals*, Mouton, Den Haag

Katz, J. (1984) *Language and other abstract objects*, Blackwell, Oxford

Kelso, J. Scott (ed.) (1982) *Human motor behavior*, Lawrence Erlbaum Associates, Hillsdale, NJ

Kimball, J. (1973) Seven principles of surface structure parsing in natural language. *Cognition, 2*, 15-47

Kiparsky, P. (1985) Some consequences of lexical phonology. *Phonology Yearbook, 2*, 83-136

Kiparsky, P. and Menn, L. (1977) On the acquisition of phonology. In

J. MacNamara (ed.), *Language learning and thought*. Academic Press, London

Lesser, R. (1978) *Linguistic investigations of aphasia*. Arnold, London

Locke, J. (1983a) Clinical phonology: the explanation and treatment of speech sound disorders. *Journal of Speech and Hearing Disorders, 48*, 339-42

Locke, J. (1983b) *Phonological acquisition and change*, Academic Press, London

McCarthy, J. (1981) The role of the evaluation metric in the acquisition of phonology. In C. Baker and J. McCarthy (eds), *The logical problem of language acquisition*, MIT Press, Cambridge, Mass.

McReynolds, L. and Engmann, D. (1975) *Distinctive feature analysis of misarticulation*, University Park Press, Baltimore

Macken, M. (1980) The child's lexical representation: the 'puzzle-puddle–pickle' evidence. *Journal of Linguistics, 16*, 1-17

Marquardt, T., Reinhart, J. and Peterson, H. (1979) Markedness analysis of phonemic substitution errors in apraxia of speech. *Journal of Communication Disorders, 12*, 481-94

Menn, L. (1978) Phonological units in beginning speech. In A. Bell and J. Hooper (eds), *Syllables and segments*, North Holland, Amsterdam, pp. 157-71.

Menn, L. (1979) Towards a psychology of phonology: child phonology as a first step. Manuscript of talk delivered to 3rd Annual Michigan State University Conference on Metatheory, Applications of Linguistics in the Human Sciences

Mohanan, K.P. (1982) *Lexical phonology*, Indiana University Linguistics Club, Bloomington

Parker, F. (1976) Distinctive features in speech pathology: phonology or phonemics? *Journal of Speech and Hearing Disorders, 41*, 23-39

Piattelli-Palmarini, M. (1980) *Language and learning*, Routledge & Kegan Paul, London

Pinker, S. (1981) Comments. In C. Baker and J. McCarthy (eds), *The logical problem of language acquisition*, MIT Press, Cambridge, Mass.

Pinker, S. (1982) A theory of the acquisition of lexical–interpretive grammars. In J. Bresnan (ed.), *The mental representation of grammatical relations*, MIT Press, Cambridge, Mass.

Pinker, S. (1984) *Language learnability and language development*, MIT Press, Cambridge, Mass.

Schmidt, R. (1976) The schema as a solution to some persistent problems in motor-learning theory. In G. Stelmach (ed.), *Motor control: issues and trends*, Academic Press, New York

Smith, N.V. (1973) *The acquisition of phonology*, Cambridge University Press, Cambridge

Smith, N.V. (1978) Lexical representations and the acquisition of phonology. In B.B. Kachru (ed.), *Linguistics in the seventies: directions and prospects. Special issue, studies in the Linguistic Sciences, vol. 8*

Spencer, A. (1986) Towards a theory of phonological development. *Lingua, 68*, 3-38

Stabler, E. (1983) How are grammars represented? *Behavioral and Brain Sciences, 6*, 391-422

Stampe, D. (1979) *A dissertation on Natural Phonology*, Garland Publishing, New York

Stelmach, G. (1978) Motor control. In K. Connolly (ed.), *Psychology surveys*, Allen & Unwin, London

Turvey, M. (1977) Preliminaries to a theory of action with reference to vision. In R. Shaw and J. Bransford (eds), *Perceiving, acting and knowing: toward an ecological psychology*, Lawrence Erlbaum Associates, Hillsdale, NJ

Waterson, N. (1971) Child phonology: a prosodic view. *Journal of Linguistics, 7*, 179-211

Waterson, N. (1987) *Prosodic phonology: the theory and its application to language acquisition and processing*, Grevatt and Grevatt, Newcastle

Weiner, F. (1979) *Phonological Process Analysis*, University Park Press, Baltimore

Weiner, F. (1984) A phonologic approach to assessment and treatment. In J. Costello (ed.), *Speech disorders in children: recent advances*, College-Hill Press, San Diego

Wexler, K. and Culicover, P. (1980) *Formal principles of language acquisition*, MIT Press, Cambridge, Mass.

White, L. (1982) *Grammatical theory and language acquistion*, Foris, Dordrecht

6

A Phonological Theory of Phonological Development

Andrew Spencer

INTRODUCTION

In this chapter I shall present in simplified outline form a theory of phonological development based on a reanalysis of the work of Smith (1973). In the interests of accessible exposition I shall not include all the technicalities of this theory and specialists in phonological theory are advised to consult Spencer (1986) for the full details. One of the practical advantages of the theory to be presented is that it does not rely as heavily as previous theories of phonological development on the writing of complex batteries of rules. While the theory is intended to be a generative theory, in many respects it appeals more to traditional phonological notions, such as the phoneme, than have earlier generative theories of phonology, and for many specialists in developmental psycholinguistics and speech pathology may well be more amenable.

Section 1.1 reviews certain important aspects of the phonological theory proposed by Chomsky and Halle (1968, henceforth *SPE*) and I then outline some of the recent (i.e. post-1975) trends in phonological theory which I believe to be of relevance for developmental phonology. These include metrical phonology (section 1.2), syllabic phonology (particularly the work of Kahn, 1976; Clements and Keyser, 1983; and Cairns and Feinstein, 1982) (section 1.3), autosegmental phonology and vowel harmony in particular (with a brief mention of McCarthy's (1979) work on non-concatenative morphology) (section 1.4), and finally in section 1.5 the notion of underspecification (Archangeli, 1984; Kiparsky, 1985).

Section 2.1 presents a brief overview of the 'classical' generative model of development, that of Smith (1973). A revision of Smith's work against the background of some of the developments discussed in section 1 is provided in section 2.2. A fairly detailed example of the kind of linguistic evidence which supports the new model is given in section 2.3.

Section 3.1 discusses some of the implications the new model has for the practising 'clinical phonologist'. I suggest that one could view the model as providing theoretical justification for adopting what in many respects is a more traditional approach to phonological analysis in the clinic. Section 3.2 considers recent work conducted by Dinnsen and his colleagues against the backdrop of the proposed model, and I indicate that certain potentially damaging but seldom remarked conceptual flaws in the popular 'phonological process analysis' approach can be remedied by adopting the stance common to the new model and the work of Dinnsen *et al.*

1. TRENDS IN PHONOLOGICAL THEORY

1.1 The *SPE* framework

The theory of generative phonology became crystallised with the publication of Chomsky and Halle (1968, known ubiquitously as '*SPE*'), one of the most influential books ever published in the field of linguistics. *SPE* encapsulated a remarkable mixture of American and European traditions (see Fischer-Jørgensen, 1975, for a history of the development of phonology, and Anderson (1985) for a somewhat more tendentious treatment of the same history), within the more general framework of generative grammar being developed at MIT, *SPE* laid the groundrules for phonological analysis (many of which still apply) but by the mid-1970s a series of results, many of them reported in unpublished MIT PhD dissertations, had questioned a number of fundamental assumptions on which the *SPE* framework rested.

I shall assume that the reader is familiar with the basic principles of generative phonology. Useful textbook treatments can be found in Schane (1973), Hyman (1975), Sommerstein (1977), and Kenstowicz and Kisseberth (1979). Hawkins (1982) contains a discussion of applications to speech pathology, and Edwards and Shriberg (1983) provide a very clear introduction to generative theory, normal phonological development and phonological disability.

The main characteristics of the *SPE* approach were the following: phonetic representations of words are derived from underlying phonological forms by a series of phonological transformational generative rules. The underlying representations (URs) take the form of strings of distinctive feature matrices, i.e. columns of distinctive features each of which characterises some phonetic property of the sound. The set of features required to characterise the sounds of the world's languages is given innately (i.e. doesn't have to be learned by the child). Most of these features are binary features (having a 'plus' or a 'minus' value), though some, like stress features, may be n-ary. In general a UR will also contain morphosyntactic (grammatical) information, since the phonological component of the grammar is preceded ('fed') by the syntactic component. One particular type of non-phonetic information the UR contains is information about morphosyntactic boundaries, of which there are three different types in *SPE*. The theory also countenances features which have no phonetic or syntactic interpretation, but are in effect instructions to apply rules in a certain fashion (or not at all). Such features, often called 'diacritics', are, for instance, used to prevent rules from applying to lexical items which exceptionally fail to undergo a rule.

The phonological rules take the form of transformations in the general case (though in practice most formulated rules are technically context-sensitive phrase structure rules). The rules map one set of representations into another by deleting, inserting or permuting segments, or changing certain feature specifications from 'plus' to 'minus' or vice-versa. The rules are given a set ordering which cannot be altered (that is, they are extrinsically ordered), though apparent reordering effects do occur, because the rules also apply in a cyclic fashion. What this means is that the rules apply to strings of feature matrices bounded on each side by morphological boundary symbols. When they have applied the innermost boundary symbols are erased, and the rules apply again from the beginning, and so on until all the boundary symbols have been erased. This principle of grammatical organisation is of supreme importance for the *SPE* analysis of stress.

The output of the set of phonological rules is a new set of

117

representations, surface representations (SRs). Very loosely speaking we may say that while URs correspond to the way words are stored SRs correspond to the way they are articulated. However, *SPE* mentions, but does not explicitly formulate, a series of rules which turn the binary feature specifications into *n*-ary specifications which reflect the precise instructions to the articulators, or equally the acoustic characteristics of the spoken form.

In the *SPE* theory every distinctive feature matrix in a UR is given a specification. However, it is well known that in many instances it is possible to predict the values of some features in a representation, either by universal principles or by language-particular principles. For instance, all sounds marked [+high] have to be marked [−low] by definition of these features. Thus, if a vowel, say, is marked [+high] in a representation, there is no need to state the feature specification for [±low]. Similarly, in English all nasals are sonorants, i.e. if a sound is marked [+nasal] it is automatically going to be marked [+sonorant]. The information in a representation which can be predicted in this fashion is referred to as redundant information (or 'a redundancy'). Redundancies also figure in the possible sequences of segments. Thus, there are no words in English which begin with three consonants whose first consonant is other than /s/. This means that once we know that a word begins with a triconsonantal cluster we can predict *all* the segmental features of the first member.

The point of giving a phoneme a representation in distinctive feature terms is to codify choices which can in principle be made in the phonetic composition of words. But this means that the *SPE* URs are in a sense misleading. To mark a nasal segment as [+sonorant] seems to imply that we can have a choice in English between such a nasal and a nasal marked [−sonorant], but this, of course, is not the case. In other words it is necessary to have some representation of words from which all the redundant information is removed, reflecting genuine choices between possible combinations of features. In *SPE* this is achieved by a set of morpheme structure conditions. There are two types of these discussed in *SPE*, the most important for our purposes being statements of the form 'If a sound has feature [αF] it has feature [βG]', or 'if a word begins with CCC the first C is /s/'. These conditions can be used to *despecify* all those feature specifications which can be predicted (which are redundant). Conventionally, a despecified feature is given the feature value '0' (also called 'blank'). A representation which includes only the unpredictable specifications is called the lexical representation.

The *SPE* model follows an influential paper of Stanley's (1967). An early approach to the problem of redundancy was to despecify redundant features at the level of the UR. Phonological rules then fell into two types: those which filled in the '0' (blank) values with appropriate '+' or '−' values (often called 'blank-filling rules') and those which changed '+' or '−' specifications into the opposite value. Stanley pointed to certain technical difficulties which arise in the *SPE* model if blank-filling rules are accepted and his proposal, which effectively outlawed such rules, was widely accepted by phonologists working within the model. This framework is shown in Figure 6.1.

Figure 6.1: The *SPE* model of phonological organisation

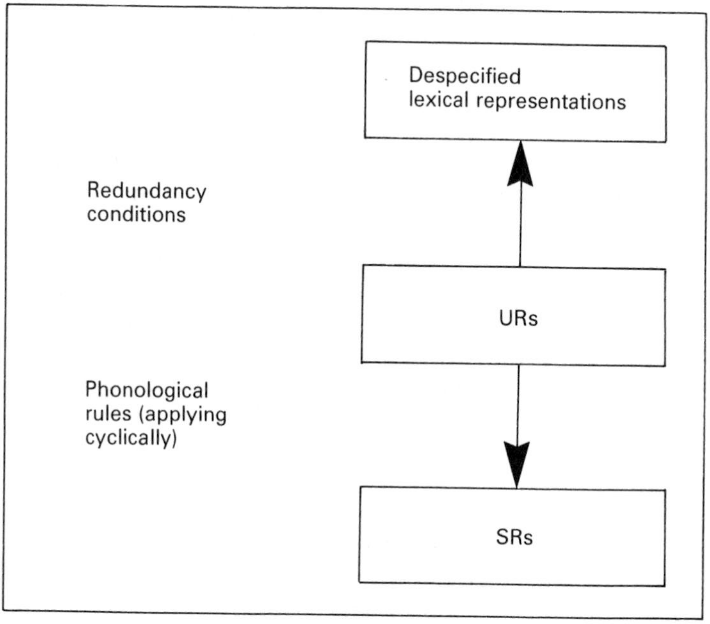

I have presented this lengthy review of the *SPE* model because (a) this forms the basis for a very influential approach

to child phonology; (b) the question of redundancy and despec-ification (or underspecification) will be important for the theory I shall describe in due course, and it is an aspect of phonological theory which tends to get neglected in textbook accounts.

1.2 Developments in post-*SPE* phonology

In the mid-1970s a series of PhD dissertations were written at MIT which had the effect of substantially altering the develop-ment of phonological theory. The initial redirection affected (a) the representation of stress systems in languages such as English (Liberman, 1975); (b) the structure of syllables (Kahn, 1976) and (c) the phonology of African tone languages (Goldsmith, 1976). In a quieter way, Paul Kiparsky and his colleagues were redefining the relationship between the phonological compo-nent of the grammar and the structure of the lexicon (i.e. the nature of lexical representations), the resulting theory coming to be known as Lexical Phonology (Kiparsky, 1982).

The first three of these new trends all had an interesting property in common. In phonological analyses within the *SPE* model phonological structures are assumed to consist of strings of segments represented as distinctive feature matrices. The only non-phonetic information in a representation is the set of boundary symbols (though these are characterised notationally in the same way as segments, using distinctive features). Unlike syntactic representations, which consist of strings of words grouped into hierarchically arranged constituents, phonological representations consist in *SPE* of linear strings. Liberman, Kahn and Goldsmith each developed theories in which phonological representations were enriched by hierarchical structures over and above the string of segments. Since phonological represent-ations now include more structure than just the linear string of segments and boundaries, such theories all tend to be called 'non-linear' ('multilinear', 'multidimensional') theories. (A good review of non-linear phonology up to 1980 is provided by van der Hulst and Smith, 1982, 1984).

Liberman formalised the notion of metrical structure in phonology. An important early published version of the theory is Liberman and Prince (1977). The theory of 'metrical phonol-ogy' which has grown out of this work is of immense signifi-cance for phonological theory. However, since it has had very little application to problems in developmental phonology I shall present only a very bare outline. An excellent, if brief, textbook description of more recent work is found in Halle and Clements (1983).

Liberman and Prince showed that a superior account of stress patterns is possible if stress is represented by binary branching trees reflecting relative prominence. A binary branching tree is simply a tree diagram all of whose nodes split into exactly two branches. Relative prominence is represented by labelling one of the two branches 's' (for 'strong') and the other 'w' (for 'weak'). This means that all such trees are combinations of the two simple trees shown in (1). This mode of representation allows us to capture the traditional idea that stress patterns are essentially rhythmic, consisting of alternating strong and weak beats.

(1)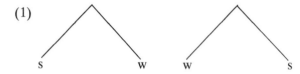

Stress rules now take the form of a series of instructions (an algorithm) for assigning that tree to a word or phrase which reflects the pattern of prominence (the main and secondary stresses). It is well known from *SPE* and earlier research that in English a great variety of complex factors condition where stress will be placed, including the number of consonants at various positions in the word, the type of consonants at the end of the word, the character of the vowels of the word and so on.

An example of how the stress pattern of an individual word can be represented is shown in (2). Examples of metrical trees representing stress in compound nouns are given in (3).

(2)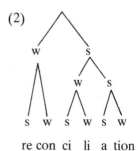

re con ci li a tion

(3a)

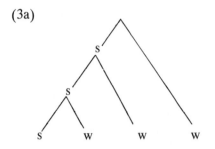

law degree requirement changes

(3b)

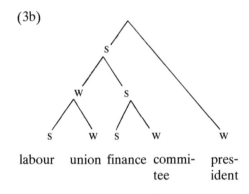

| labour | union | finance | commi-tee | pres-ident |

1.3 Syllabic phonology

Kahn introduced the notion of the syllable into generative phonology (in *SPE* it was possible to identify syllables but the notion played no direct role in the theory), and he showed that generalisations would be missed if phonological rules couldn't refer directly to syllable structure. (In this respect he was prefigured by, for instance, Anderson and Jones, 1974 and Hooper, 1972.)

SPE makes no reference to syllables (except for a famous oblique allusion, p. 241 fn. 3), it being assumed that the notion 'syllable' can always be reconstructed, and that it is thus superfluous. Subsequent work suggested this was wrong (Fudge, 1969; Hooper, 1972, 1976; Venneman, 1972; Anderson and Jones, 1974). Kahn's dissertation provided extensive justification of the view that phonological descriptions must be permitted to refer to syllables and parts of syllables in order to capture linguistically significant generalisations. Kahn claimed a grammar must have rules specifying how syllables are constructed, and that they interact with other phonological rules such as aspiration of initial plosives in English.

Every language permits syllables of certain types and rejects syllables of other types. Some only allow so-called 'open syllables' consisting only of a vowel or consonant plus vowel (CV), and reject consonant clusters or closed syllables (i.e. syllables ending in a consonant, CVC). Others permit syllables with extremely complex clusters initially or finally (Russian, for example, has words like /mtsensk/, /lakomstf/, /vzgljat/). English allows initial clusters of certain kinds but not others, for instance /tr-/ is a common cluster but /tl-/ is impossible.

One problem facing the student of the syllable is knowing where one syllable ends and the next begins when a cluster occurs word-medially. A common approach has been to split up such clusters in such a way as to minimise the cluster at the end of the first syllable and maximise the cluster at the beginning ('onset') of the following syllable. This is known as the Maximal Onset Principle. Thus, we can syllabify a word such as 'restrain' as in (4a) and 'extra' as in (4b) (where the dot indicates the syllable boundary).

(4a) ri . strein   (4b) ek . stra

This still leaves a problem with a word like 'phoneme': should this be (5a) or (5b)? One traditional answer (justified in some detail by Anderson and Jones, 1974) was to say that the medial segment belonged simultaneously to the end of the first and the beginning of the second syllable, in other words that the /n/ in (5) is 'ambisyllabic'.

(5a) fo . nim   (5b) fon . im

Kahn utilised a format developed by Goldsmith (see below) to represent syllable structure, one of whose advantages is that it permits a neat characterisation of ambisyllabicity. Given a string of segments, syllabication rules first link a 'syllable' node (S) to the vowels ('syllabic nuclei'), then link each such node to preceding consonants, respecting the language's constraints on syllable-initial clusters (this incorporates the Maximal Onset principle), and then does the same for the end of the syllable. Finally, except in very careful speech styles, a further rule links the first consonant of a syllable with the preceding vowel, making that consonant ambisyllabic. A sample derivation is provided in (6).

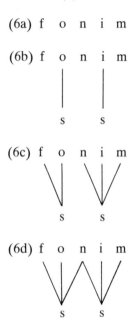

(6a) f o n i m

(6b) f o n i m
     s   s

(6c) f o n i m
     s   s

(6d) f o n i m
     s   s

Kahn's theory has been put to good use to uncover the patterns in the speech of a phonologically disordered child by Gandour (1981); the first example of the application of non-linear phonological theory to child language.

In Kahn's theory syllables are given a very simple hierarchical structure. A slightly more elaborate version of this structure has been described by Clements and Keyser (1983). They observe that phonological rules seem to refer to three aspects of structure: syllables, consonant/vowel strings and segments themselves. It is quite common for languages to have rules which affect the basic 'skeleton' of Cs and Vs in a word without caring what phonemes those Cs and Vs are. For instance, we find rules deleting the final consonant of a word-final two-membered cluster, or inserting a consonant (e.g. a glide) between two adjacent vowels *irrespective of the nature of those consonants or vowels*. Therefore, a more economical description of the facts will often be possible if we are allowed to refer solely to the CV skeleton (or template). In a multidimensional theory of phonology this means that the segmental specification of a sound (e.g. its specification for features such as [nasal] [high], etc.) can be thought of as occupying one dimension of the representation, and the sequence of Cs and Vs (or CV slots) another dimension. These dimensions are generally referred to as *tiers*. The Clements and Keyser theory is known as 'three-tiered' or 'CV phonology'.

While the CV phonology approach to the syllable has not been explicitly applied to child language the notion of a separate CV tier or skeleton figures prominently in the theory developed in Spencer (1986). It has been widely accepted that there is the need to distinguish a separate CV tier since the pioneering work of McCarthy (1979, 1981) on so-called 'non-concatenative' morphological systems. Moreover, McCarthy's work shows that it is frequently necessary to refer separately to the consonantism and the vocalism in a phonological representation. An introduction to McCarthy's ideas can be found in Halle and Clements (1983) and in van der Hulst and Smith (1982), and a brief presentation of his analysis set in the context of child phonology is given in Spencer (1984). It is sufficient to say here that it is crucial to the theory of development presented in Spencer (1986) that rules be able to refer separately to C slots or V slots, systematically ignoring the other type of slot.

The theories of Kahn, and of Clements and Keyser, both assign a 'flat' structure to the syllable. That is, a syllable is for them, a string of elements (phonemes or CV slots), it doesn't have any richer hierarchical structure. This means that in tree diagrams there are no nodes intervening between the lowest (CV) level (or tier) and the syllable node (though Clements and Keyser do suggest the need to distinguish the syllable nucleus). However, it has often been assumed that syllables can be broken up into smaller constituents which are nonetheless larger than single segments. In (7) we see a diagram of such a richer conception of the syllable.

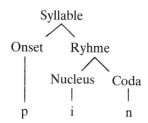

Diagrams such as this are reminiscent of phrase markers for syntax, and some phonologists believe that formal descriptive apparatus borrowed from syntactic theory can elucidate syllable structure. A good example of this line of reasoning is provided by Cairns and Feinstein (1982). They use the notion 'head' (i.e. the obligatory member of a constituent) to characterise the syllable and its constituents. In a case such as 'sprint', for instance, one might propose a diagram such as (8), where 'H' stands for 'head of a constituent'. In (8) the nucleus would be the head of the rhyme, and the rhyme would be the head of the syllable. Similarly, the /p/ would be the head of the onset. (Cairns and Feinstein actually remain agnostic about the precise structure of codas).

(8)

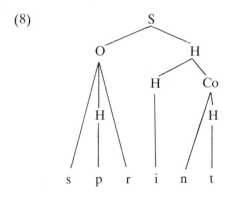

I make use of the Cairns and Feinstein theory of syllable structure in my reanalysis of Smith's work (Spencer, 1986), but it will be some time before the dust settles on syllable theory, and it is as yet quite unclear what form the best theory will take. However, many of the 'processes' commonly described in the child language literature are syllable structure processes, and we can be fairly confident that a much better understanding of child phonology would result from a more serious consideration of the role of syllable structure in developing systems.

1.4 Autosegmental phonology

Structuralist theories of phonology concentrated primarily on the nature of phonemic contrasts and devoted relatively little attention to phonological processes above the level of the segment ('suprasegmental' processes, sometimes called 'prosodic' processes). An interesting exception was the London (Firthian) School of Prosodic Phonology, which concentrated much of its attention on precisely such phenomena. In generative phonology, however, it was not until the work of Goldsmith that the idea of suprasegmental processes was taken seriously.

Goldsmith's main research effort was devoted to tone patterns in African languages. He developed the idea that the tone 'melody' of a word is independent of the segmental composition of the word, inasmuch as there are phonological processes which affect one dimension but not the other. In the interests of exposition I shall illustrate the basic ideas of Goldsmith's thesis with examples from English intonation (cf. Liberman and Pierrehumbert, 1984; Gussenhoven, 1983, for genuine attempts at such a treatment). The example is a little artificial in that the tonal phenomena Goldsmith looked at generally induced grammatical or lexical meaning differences.

Let us imagine that the intonation contour of an English phrase consists of tunes characterised as sequences of high and low tones. The standard falling intonation can then be regarded as a high tone followed by a low tone (HL). There is a tune in English, however, which is more complex than this in that it comprises a HLH contour. It signals a question or a surprised statement, and would normally be found on an utterance such as (9) with main emphasis on 'Tom'.

(9) Did *Tom* put the cat out?

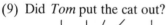
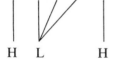

Ignoring for the moment the fact that the second H tone is lower than the first, and various other subtleties, we can give a fairly complete characterisation of the intonation contour once we have specified the tonal 'melody' (HLH) and the place where each tone movement takes place.

If we associate the tones with different words we get a different type of utterance, though we are still clearly using the same intonation contour. Examples (10) show what happens if we put the main emphasis on 'cat' or 'out'.

(10a)Did Tom put the *cat* out?

H LH

(10b)Did Tom put the cat *out*?

HLH

In (10a) we have a compound tone on the word 'out', moving from low to high. In (10b) all the pitch movement is located on a single word. Sentence (11) is another example of the same phenomenon.

(11) Me?!

HLH

What these examples illustrate in a very crude way is that we can regard the intonational tune and the string of segments making up the sentence as separate entities, from the point of view of phonology. The tune remains the same in examples (9)–(11); what changes is the segmental composition of the sentences, or, in the case of (9, 10), the manner in which the tune is *associated* to the segment string. In other words, we again see evidence that phonological representations must be multidimensional, in the sense that we must separate the segmental 'tier' from the tonal 'tier'. Since we are regarding tones as very much like autonomous segments existing on their own 'tier', Goldsmith coined the term 'autosegmental' for such representations. Each of the tones is then an 'autosegment'.

We can also see that an important aspect of this distinction is that differences in phonological representations can be the result of a difference in the way that elements of one tier are associated with elements of another. In the diagrams I have drawn so far (including the representations of syllabic structure) I have represented association simply by drawing lines. This is the notational convention established by Goldsmith. He showed that much of the patterning of tonal systems he studied could be understood by imposing tight restrictions on the manner in which such association is effected. He hypothesised that certain universal conventions govern association, and he referred to these collectively as the Well-Formedness Condition. The precise wording of this condition is still disputatious, but one principle has remained sacrosanct to date; namely, that in drawing diagrams with association lines, the association lines are not allowed to cross each other. Perhaps surprisingly, by imposing this restriction it is possible to rule out of the theory a large number of possible tone systems which don't in fact occur. This means that the theory can help explain why it is that only certain patterns are found.

An enormous amount of research has subsequently been devoted to the autosegmental analysis of tone systems (cf., for example, the papers in Clements and Goldsmith, 1985), testifying to the value of this approach to the problem of tone. However, the basic principles of autosegmental phonology have proved invaluable for other phenomena too. The syllabication rules of Kahn, and of Clements and Keyser, are essentially autosegmental. Moreover, following the work of Clements (1980, first written 1976) considerable efforts have been expended on providing autosegmental analyses of long-distance assimilation processes, notably vowel harmony. This is of great importance for students of child phonology because such long-distance assimilations (especially in the form of consonant harmony) are characteristic of early articulation.

Many languages of the world impose constraints on the kinds of vowels which may co-occur within a word or even a phrase. A typical example is Finnish. This language has the vowel phoneme inventory given in (12).

(12) i   y   u

      e   ø   o

      æ   a

Disregarding the vowels /i,e/, which are 'neutral', these vowels are distributed according to a rule of vowel harmony which states that either all the vowels in a word are [−back] (/y, ø, æ/) or they are [+back] (/u,o,a/). Finnish is a highly inflecting language with a great many suffixes. Most of these appear in two forms, with either a front vowel form or a back vowel form depending on whether the stem to which the suffix attaches has front or back vowels. For instance, the suffix -ssa/-ssæ means 'in, on'. Its use is illustrated in (13).

(13a) talo 'house' talossa 'in the house'
(13b) pøydæ 'table' pøydæssæ 'on the table'

The autosegmental approach to harmony systems relies on two ideas. First, the [back] feature is an autosegment, existing on its own level distinct from the segmental tier. Second, each of the vowels of a word is 'underspecified' in lexical or underlying representation with respect to that autosegment. A phonological derivation mapping the underlying representation into the surface (pronounced) form includes a principle by which the autosegment is associated with each of the vowels in the word. Let A, U, O represent the vowels /a,æ/ /u,y/ /o,ø/ unspecified for the feature [back]. This means that we can represent the vowels /a/ and /æ/ as (14a,b) respectively.

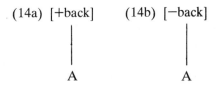

The underlying representations of the words of (13) will be (15). Derivations are illustrated in (16). The dotted line means 'gets associated to'. The convention (which is often significant in more complex cases) is the association proceeds from left to right until all the vowels have been associated with the autosegment.

(15a) [+back]   [+back]

   tAlO   tAlOssA

(15b) [−back]   [−back]

   pOUdA   pOUdAssA

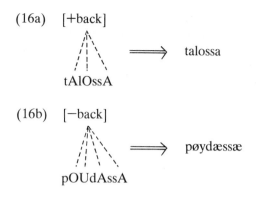

(16a)   [+back]

tAlOssA $\implies$ talossa

(16b)   [−back]

pOUdAssA $\implies$ pøydæssæ

1.5. Underspecification

I mentioned in section 1.1 that *SPE* rejected the idea that lexical redundancies were extracted from phonological underlying representations, and adopted the convention that they were captured by conditions on lexical representations. Thus, in a phonological derivation the starting point, the phonological UR, is always fully specified for all its features. The astute reader will have noticed from previous discussion that this view is already challenged by non-linear approaches to phonology. For instance, in discussing Finnish vowel harmony we noted that the starting point for the phonological derivation (i.e. the UR) contained vowels which were not fully specified for the feature [back]. In a more subtle way the rules which assign syllable structure and metrical stress structure can be thought of as providing structure which is not specified in the UR. In recent work within the framework of lexical phonology (Kiparsky, 1982, 1985) it is assumed that all redundancy is extracted from URs (much as in the theory of Halle, 1959) and that blank-filling (structure-building) rules contribute to the phonological derivation. A representation in which all redundant feature values are replaced by blanks (zeros) is called 'underspecified'. A systematic exposition of a theory relying on underspecification is the doctoral dissertation of Archangeli (1984).

The motivation for the technicalities surrounding current conceptions of underspecification is sometimes theory-internal, aimed, for example, at meeting the technical objections levelled by Stanley (1967) at earlier versions of the idea. However, to understand how underspecification can be useful in developing

131

a theory of the acquisition of articulation it will be necessary to touch briefly on the mechanics of Archangeli's system.

Suppose we have an underlying vowel phoneme inventory consisting of the five cardinals. These can be defined by the distinctive feature matrix of (17) using the features [high, low, back, round].

(17)

	i	e	a	o	u
high	+	−	−	−	+
low	−	−	+	−	−
back	−	−	+	+	+
round	−	−	−	+	+

If, however, we simply wish to keep each phoneme separate from the others we can ignore certain specifications as redundant. We know, of course, that the feature specification [−low] is redundant for /i,u/ (recall that all [+high] segments are by definition [−low]). Similarly, given that /a/ is [+low] the specification [−high] is redundant for this vowel. However, given this inventory we can also say that provided we know that a sound is [+round] we also know that it must be [+back]. This is another way of saying that there are no front-rounded sounds (such as /y,ø/) in this inventory. This is not a matter of universal definition. Front-rounded sounds occur in many languages (e.g. Finnish), but not in the inventory of (17). We can therefore say that round vowels are redundantly specified for the feature [back].

Pursuing this logic we could arrive at the matrix in (18). Zero specification is represented by a blank space.

(18)

	i	e	a	o	u
high	+	−		−	+
low					
back	−	−	+		
round	−	−	−	+	+

This is not the only possible such matrix; in general there will be several different ways of underspecifying a matrix. I choose this one for illustrative purposes. One of the things it illustrates is that the feature [low] might be regarded as completely redundant. The only [+low] sound, /a/, also happens to be the only [+back, −round] sound, so knowing the latter feature set we can predict the value of [low]. Alternatively, of course, we can predict that a sound will be [+back, −round] (and, of course, [−high]) given that it is [+low]. It is this kind of reciprocity which ensures that we often have a choice of how to underspecify. However, Archangeli (1984) adopts the principle that the fewer features you need to define the matrix as a whole the better; so that if we can find an underspecification which rids us of certain features altogether, this is to be preferred. If we still have a choice we select the underspecification which uses fewest positive or negative specifications (i.e. which has the greatest number of blanks).

To reconstitute matrix (17) from (18) we assume a set of redundancy rules which take the shape of (19) (Archangeli refers to these as Default Rules).

$$(19) \quad [\ ] \Rightarrow [+\text{back}] \ / \begin{bmatrix} \underline{\hspace{2cm}} \\ +\text{round} \end{bmatrix}$$

Matrix (18) is essentially the kind of matrix to be found in early generative phonologies. Archangeli introduces a subtle twist into the argument by noticing that (18) still contains redundant information. Recall that all features are binary, having values either '+' or '−'. Suppose for a given feature we decide that one of these values will be the 'marked' value, and the other the 'unmarked' value. Then rather than marking some segments '+' and others '−' for a given feature we can adopt the convention that we only indicate segments bearing the marked value; all the other segments have values either given by redundancy rules such as (19) or given by a set of conventional Complement Rules which simply state that, if a blank specification isn't filled in by a Default Rule then it is given the unmarked value for that feature. This implies that the Complement Rules have to apply after the relevant Default Rules. This is because there is nothing to guarantee that the value assigned by the Default Rule and that assigned by the Complement Rule will be the same. By virtue of a general (universal) convention on rule application (the 'elsewhere condition' — see Kiparsky, 1982, for a recent statement of this) the Default Rule will always win the race with a Complement Rule.

If we let marked values for our remaining features be [+high, +back, +round] we end up with matrix (20). Notice that one of the vowels (/e/) has no specifications at all; it is the maximally underspecified segment (given this underspecification). Notice also that it is not possible to distinguish these five segments with any fewer specifications. One segment has no marks at all, three are distinguished by only one mark and one segment bears two marks. We need at least three binary features to distinguish five segments, and it should be clear that three segments and five marks is the maximum degree of underspecification we could achieve in principle.

(20)

	i	e	a	o	u
high	+			+	
back			+		
round				+	+

There are other technicalities surrounding the notion of underspecification and it should be admitted that in many respects the details of this approach to phonology are more controversial than the details of the non-linear theories I have described. Nonetheless, some variety of underspecification is current in almost all contemporary models of generative phonology.

2. CURRENT PHONOLOGICAL THEORY AND THE DEVELOPMENT OF ARTICULATION

In this section I shall briefly review what we may regard as the 'classical' generative theory of the acquisition of phonology, and then develop a more contemporary viewpoint on the basis of the trends in phonological theory described in section 1.

2.1. The 'classical' theory

One of the most detailed, carefully argued and influential pieces of research on child phonology was Smith's (1973) analysis of the speech of his son, Amahl, between the ages of roughly two and four years. Smith analysed his data within the *SPE* framework, providing a thoroughly explicit rule system for the initial stage that he observed, and showing how that rule system changed with development.

Smith adopted the *SPE* assumption that a phonological

system consists of a set of URs (underlying representations), a set of SRs (surface representations), and a set of phonological rules mapping the former into the latter. Now, when a phonologist analyses a new language for the first time he is given the SRs (these are very roughly what he gets when he writes down words in broad transcription) but he does not know the rules or the URs. Obviously, these are interlinked in that if the UR postulated by the linguist is wrong, he will have to write wrong rules to map it onto the SR. On the other hand, even if he hits upon the right UR he still has to make sure he is using a correctly formulated rule. Writing a phonology is then a trial-and-error process, subject to continual revision and improvement.

If Smith had had to figure out Amahl's URs as well as his rule system his task would have been truly Herculean. Fortunately he was able to make an assumption which simplified the problem. From a very early age normal children can correctly distinguish similar but different words in their language even if they can't say them, or even if they neutralise the pronunciation difference in their own speech. Thus, while many children would pronounce the words 'lolly' and 'lorry' identically, they don't usually confuse the terms when they are used by others. Smith hypothesised that even before the child begins to speak properly he has figured out the surface representations of the adult form of common words (with a handful of interesting exceptions); that is, he can assign a fully specified feature matrix to all such words. However, his production doesn't reflect this perfect perceptual competence. Smith therefore claimed that the adult SRs served as the child's URs and that the child developed a rule system for simplifying these URs into his own SRs. Smith called these phonologial rules 'realisation rules'. The model is shown in figure 6.2.

Figure 6.2: The 'classical' model of child phonology (Smith, 1973)

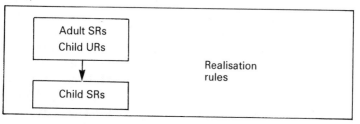

This model assumes that the child never makes any perceptually based errors in analysing the incoming adult SRs. Subsequent research (e.g. Macken, 1980) has shown that this is not quite correct, though it remains essentially true for normal children. In a later version of the model, therefore, Smith inserts a perceptual filter between adult SRs and child URs to reflect such misstorage.

Smith's model has two considerable merits. It is justified by essentially linguistic data and argumentation and it is maximally simple, in that it does not posit any apparatus over and above what is essential for getting the facts straight, given the linguistic framework of analysis which Smith adopts. One could, of course, quarrel with Smith's choice of the then new *SPE* framework, but Smith's reply would be 'what superior framework is there?'.

Given the changes that have taken place in phonological theory, we could reply to this hypothetical question by saying 'the theoretical proposals outlined in section 1'. In other words, we could see what the consequences would be of taking Smith's data, treating them like any other set of linguistic data, and analysing them in the way such data are customarily analysed by contemporary phonologists. One important justification for this exercise is that many of the phenomena of child language, i.e. syllable structure processes, consonant harmonies, reduplication processes and so on, are precisely the phenomena which the *SPE* model handled rather badly, and for which the recent theories have been developed. In the next subsection I discuss some such cases in more detail.

2.2. A non-linear model of development

I begin my reanalysis of Smith's data with a phenomenon known as 'lateral harmony'. Smith reports that if a word consisted solely of liquids or glides one of which was /l/ then Amahl pronounced all the consonants in the word as /l/. Thus, 'lorry' was pronounced just like 'lolly' while 'yellow' was pronounced /lelo/. A phonologist quickly recognises this as a case of bidirectional harmony defined over the feature [lateral]. This is the same type of harmony we saw with Finnish vowels. Smith wrote a somewhat complex set of rules which generate the lateral harmony data. These rules resemble in many respects the sort of rules which some phonologists wrote within the *SPE* framework for cases such as Finnish vowel harmony. Many of the criticisms which adherents of non-linear phonology levelled against the *SPE* linear approaches to vowel harmony apply to Smith's account.

In a non-linear account of lateral harmony we would simply assume that URs containing liquids and glides are underspecified for the feature [lateral]. If the word contains a lateral somewhere then the word is provided with an autosegment [+lateral]. Otherwise, it is given the autosegment [−lateral]. Thus, the words 'yellow' and 'yo-yo' would be given representations such as (21).

(21a) [+lateral]   (21b) [−lateral]

$$\begin{bmatrix} C \\ +son \\ -nas \end{bmatrix} e \quad \begin{bmatrix} C \\ +son \\ -nas \end{bmatrix} o \qquad \begin{bmatrix} C \\ +son \\ -nas \end{bmatrix} o \quad \begin{bmatrix} C \\ +son \\ -nas \end{bmatrix} o$$

A phonological derivation then consists very simply of linking the [lateral] autosegment to the C slots. Notice that in the theory of autosegmental phonology this would not be a rule in the child's system; rather it would be a universal convention about how to interpret representations such as (21). This account is vastly simpler than Smith's rule (cf. discussion in Spencer, 1986, pp. 8 ff.).

Suppose we accept the above argument and adopt an autosegmental analysis of lateral harmony. How does this affect our more general assumptions? Recall that a crucial element of the autosegmental analysis to harmony is that the harmonising elements (the liquids and glides in our example) are *underspecified* for the harmonic feature (i.e. [lateral]). But in the *SPE* model assumed by Smith there is no underspecification of URs. This might not be too damaging, except that Smith assumes that the child's URs are identical to the adult SRs, and adult SRs are always fully specified matrices on anybody's theory.

If we wished to retain the parsimony of Smith's model we could try assuming that the child can only perceive part of the adult SR; namely that it has liquids and glides and that one of them is a lateral in some words. In some cases of pathological development, as well as some cases of normal development, something of this sort seems to happen. Indeed, it is the reason that Smith was compelled to concede a (limited) perceptual filter for normal development. However, in the present case it seems that Amahl had no difficulty perceiving the difference between 'lorry' and 'lolly'.

This means that we must assume a model in which there is an extra level of linguistic representation. We have to retain Smith's box marked 'Child UR' (and his perceptual filter, of course), and this will reflect the contrasts and phonological relationships the child correctly perceives. We also retain his box marked 'Child SR' — this needn't change. But we also need an extra level intervening between the old 'Child UR' and the 'Child SR' boxes. This extra box will contain the URs such as (21) which contain underspecified segments. Let us call the old 'Child UR' box the child's 'input representations' (or IRs) and the new box the child's 'output underlying representations' or OPURs.

We also need to relate these three boxes. The simplest assumption is that the IRs are fully specified and that the OPURs are derived from the IRs by simply despecifying certain feature values in accordance with the child's own phonological system. In practice it turns out to be simpler (in the case of younger children) to state which feature values aren't despecified and then despecify the rest with one rule (cf. Spencer, 1986, p. 16). Let us call the processes which determine which of the OPUR features are specified and which not 'realisation processes'. We now have a way of deriving a set of underspecified underlying representations for the child's output. All that remains is to respecify the underspecified features in accordance with the child's phonology. This we can do with a set of rules mapping OPURs to child SRs which I shall call 'pronunciation rules'. The entire model is presented in Figure 6.3.

The sceptical reader may feel we have got rather a lot of mileage out of one very simple example. However, the example is far from isolated. Moreover, we must remember that the model of child phonology we adopt is crucially dependent on the model of phonology we adopt. Smith was able to account for Amahl's system by appealing to no more than URs and SRs in the child's system, solely because he assumed (with *SPE*) that all URs are fully specified. As soon as any form of underspecification is assumed, the 'two boxes' model will have to be

Figure 6.3

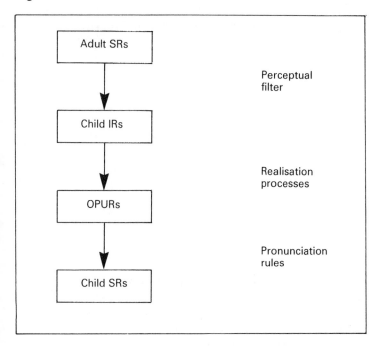

abandoned, because there will have to be an extra box containing the underspecified representations.

However, if we make use of other post-*SPE* developments we encounter further evidence to support the distinction between IRs and OPURs. It is well known that many children have processes which affect syllable structure in a systematic way. Amahl, for instance, only allowed very simple syllables in his early speech, no more complex than CVC. Some children pass through lengthy initial stages of development in which they only permit open (CV) syllables and this 'open syllable syndrome' is a frequently encountered phenomenon in speech therapy clinics. I argue in Spencer (1986, pp. 12 ff.) that Amahl's syllable structure can be understood extremely simply on the basis of Figure 6.3. If we assume that Amahl's syllable structure at the IR level is that of the adult form we can account for his output syllable structure by assuming a simple realisation process. This process matches the IR form (i.e. the adult word) to a simple template, which is represented in (22). It will be clear that I am assuming the theory of syllable structure offered by Cairns and Feinstein (1982). However, as far as I can tell, similar results could be obtained with any decent theory of the syllable, provided the rules were altered accordingly.

(22)

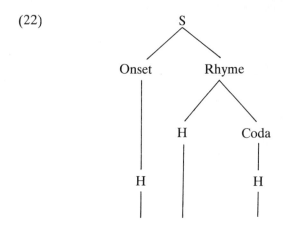

This is to be interpreted as follows: the realisation process acts as a filter on syllable structure by deleting all parts of a syllable except the head of the rhyme (i.e. the syllable nucleus or peak, the V of the CVC sequence), the head of the onset and the head of the coda. Such deletion can be thought of as an extreme form of despecification. As can be seen from (23) this means that the OPUR for a word such as 'stroke' will be //touk//.

(23)

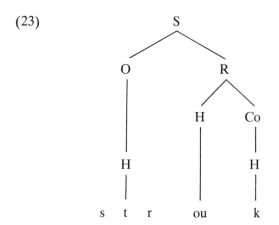

To achieve the same results in the *SPE* framework (or any of the 'phonological process analysis' frameworks) we would have to assume a fairly complicated battery of rules deleting segments of a particular type in particular environments ordered extrinsically with respect to other rules. However, there is an important empirical advantage to an approach such as this. I shall describe this in the next subsection.

2.3. Labial attraction and the development of syllable structure

I characterised realisation processes as processes which despecified all but a number of features effectively coding the fact that the child makes fewer contrasts in his output than he is capable of discriminating on the input side. However, realisation processes have to be more sophisticated than a simple filter admitting some contrasts but not others. In the case of lateral harmony, for instance, I argued that the child 'knows' on the output side that a word with liquids and glides does or doesn't contain a lateral, but doesn't 'know' where the lateral is. I represented this idea by assuming an OPUR with underspecified consonants and a [lateral] autosegment. But this means that the [lateral] autosegment must survive the filter function of the realisation processes. Thus one of our realisation processes must 'float' the autosegment from lexical representations rather than merely despecifying it.

Another phonological process in Amahl's speech necessitates a more complex realisation process. Words beginning with a Cw cluster and ending in a consonant, such as 'quick', 'queen', or 'twice', were subject to a process by which the labiality of the /w/ was absorbed by the final consonant, while the /w/ itself (along with all postconsonantal sonorants) was deleted. I have called this process 'labial attraction'. Thus, 'quick' was pronounced /kip/, 'queen', /ki:m/. This process didn't affect words beginning with /sw-/ clusters, however. Smith accounted for this patterning by assuming

(i)   a rule deleting /s/ at the beginning of a cluster;
(ii) a rule assimilating the labial features of /w/ in a Cw cluster to the following consonant;
(iii) a rule deleting postconsonantal sonorants (including, of course, the tokens of /w/ which had triggered the assimilation under (ii)).

These rules had to be extrinsically ordered with respect to each other. Sample derivations are provided in (24).

(24a) swi:t ('sweet')   (24b) kwik ('quick')
   (i) Ø   —
   (ii) —   p
   (iii) —   Ø

output wi:t   kip

In (24a) rule (i) 'bleeds' rule (ii) since the /w/ is no longer part of a Cw cluster.

In the current theory we would explain these phenomena differently. Rule (ii) would remain in essence, except that we would assume that the OPUR included a [labial] autosegment and that a specific rule attached this autosegment to the last consonant of the syllable. (The technicalities of underspecification mean that the result will automatically be a /p/ or /m/ without the need for further rules, but I skip these subtleties). Rules (i) and (iii), however, are an automatic consequence of the operation of the syllabic template, given natural assumptions about the structure of syllables. The most reasonable way of regarding /sw/ clusters is to treat the /s/ as a peripheral, non-obligatory part of the cluster (onset) (this is more obvious in the case of three-membered clusters such as /skw/). This means that /w/ must be the head of the onset in /sw/ clusters. On the other hand in obstruent + sonorant clusters (such as /kw/) it is equally clear that it is the obstruent that is the head. Therefore, the syllable template will have the effect of simultaneously deleting cluster initial /s/ and postconsonantal /w/. However, we must code the fact that in words such as 'quick' the child knows on the output side that there is a labial element somewhere (i.e. he must have the [labial] autosegment in his OPUR). This means that the realisation process effecting syllable structure simplification must be made slightly more complex: when it filters out 'postconsonantal' sonorants it must 'float' the labial feature from Cw clusters, just as another realisation process must float a [lateral] autosegment. In the present case the realisation process need be sensitive only to occurrences of [+labial].

A 'derivation' for the words 'sweet' and 'quick' is given in (25) and (26).

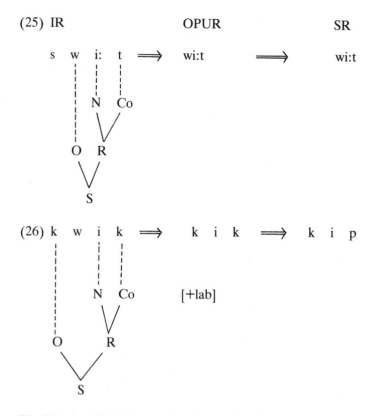

(25) IR   OPUR   SR

The history of labial attraction is very interesting. One day, Amahl suddenly announced 'Daddy, I can say [kwik]' and was able immediately to pronounce all other such words (e.g. 'queen' and 'twice') (Smith 1973, p. 65). Within the *SPE* framework there is simply no way of stating formally that the labial attraction rule is lost because the postconsonantal sonorant deletion rule is lost (as the reader can ascertain by checking Smith's rules). This is an important observation because it demonstrates an explanatory inadequacy in Smith's framework.

An interesting aspect of these derivations is that the explanation of labial attraction hinges crucially on the formulation of the realisation rule which accounts for syllable structure. As the child's phonology develops, his realisation rules effect fewer and less drastic changes. In particular the syllable template becomes more complex as a greater variety and complexity of syllable types is pronounced correctly. Consider what happens when the syllable template changes so as to accept clusters of obstruent +

143

sonorant. This means that the realisation process which has the effect of deleting /w/ but leaving behind the [+labial] autosegment will no longer operate. This means that the [+labial] autosegment will no longer appear in OPURs and hence that no linking of that autosegment to the next consonant will occur. In other words the child's pronunciation will jump straight from /kip/ to /kwik/ with no intervening form such as /kwip/. This, of course, is precisely what happened. It is a natural consequence of the formalism adopted here, but is impossible to state in Smith's rule system. It is the kind of linguistic evidence which weighs heavily in favour of the analysis involving non-linear representations and against the linear account.

3. SOME IMPLICATIONS FOR THE ANALYSIS OF PHONOLOGICAL DISABILITY

3.1. Practical analysis

In section 2.1 I pointed out that, working within an *SPE* framework, Smith was able to simplify the job of the analyst by assuming that the child's UR is identical to the adult SR. This means that all the analyst need do is work out rules which take URs into SRs. He doesn't have the additional burden of the 'real' linguist of figuring out the URs themselves. Smith's assumption is shared by Stampe (1979) and subsequent investigators who have described the analysis of 'phonological processes' (e.g. Ingram, 1976). The assumption is partially retained in the new model of development I have offered. The input representations are identical to Smith's Child URs (I follow Smith, of course, in assuming some kind of perceptual filter to handle the cases Macken (1980) discusses).

However, it is no longer the case that the analyst knows what the equivalent of a phonological underlying representation is, simply on the basis of knowing the adult SR. In order to establish the form of OPURs (and hence the nature of the realisation processes and the pronunciation rules) the analyst must behave just like a linguist confronted with a new language. S/he must establish an output phoneme inventory for the child, and a set of phonotactics (including canonical syllable structure). In point of fact, since the OPUR level bears a special relationship to the IR level this task is actually slightly more straightforward than that of the field linguist. Nonetheless, far less can be taken for granted than on the older model.

Despite this, there are respects in which the new model makes it easier to analyse developing phonologies. Since many of the rules and processes of the classical model are replaced by single templates one need simply state 'the canonical syllable structure is such-and-such', and 'the realisation processes transmit the following aspects of adult syllable structure', and nothing more need be said. In particular, it is usually the case that the analyst doesn't have to worry about writing rules in the correct order (because there is only one rule!). S/he therefore doesn't have to puzzle over conundrums such as what it means for a child to order his phonological processes and how you get a child in therapy to apply his processes in a different order.

One of the useful features of underspecification theory is that it allows the analyst to make use of the traditional phoneme concept without having to provide the complex batteries of rules required in the classical model. This is because many of the feature specifications are provided by Complement Rules or Default Rules, and these are probably not crucial to a gross understanding of the child's system. As far as the segmental phonology of the child is concerned what the clinician is more interested in is the set of contrasts the child can make. On the current model this can be established by simply working out the child's output phoneme inventory at the level of OPURs. Using, say, a phonological process analysis framework (which to all intents and purposes is a simplified version of the classical model) this information could only be gleaned by determining whether the process (or its developmental variant) applied to a greater or lesser number of input forms, and even then the calculation would be equivocal.

Establishing the child's phoneme inventory is not sufficient in itself, of course, to characterise a child's progress. Syllable/word structure development is extremely important. In the classical, linear, model such information is inevitably hidden away in syllable structure processes, which makes it very difficult to see how the child's system is progressing. If a child who drops all final consonants, say, starts producing them, then we can, admittedly, say that the child has simply lost a process, and that this constitutes improved articulation. In many cases, however, the process simply changes (often becoming more complex in its statement) and the significance of this for the child's development is often very opaque.

Adopting a non-linear framework allows us to fractionate segmental and syllable structure information, for our theory invokes representations in which they appear on different tiers or dimensions. The practical advantage of this is that the current model licenses separate examination of segment and syllable structure, whereas this would technically be an error in the linear framework. Just such a separation is found useful in a profiling system such as PROP (Crystal, 1982). The recent rediscovery of syllable structure by generative phonology has meant that phonologists (including clinical phonologists) are now able to investigate differences between the constituents of a syllable, particularly the main constituents of onset and rhyme. I mentioned Kahn's researches into the properties of ambisyllabic consonants and the insightful way this has been applied to disordered phonology by Gandour (1981). What this means is that it makes good sense on the current model to begin an analysis of child data by looking at segments in word-initial position (where we will find just onsets), word-final position (where we will find just codas), and word-medial position (where we will find consonants which are both codas and onsets, i.e. ambisyllabic consonants). Clinicians will recognise that this approach is eminently compatible with traditional practice.

Another advantage of the current perspective is that it provides a way of investigating word structure. Children often pass through phases in which words conform to a canonical CV structure, a simple and typical example being the strategy of reduplication. A case of exactly this sort in the clinical literature is analysed in Spencer (1984). Phenomena of this kind are particularly difficult to describe elegantly within the classical model (especially in the Phonological Process Analysis variant).

It may appear from the foregoing that there is little left of Phonological Process Analysis (which is, as I have said, basically a highly simplified version of Smith's classical model). However, although many of the phenomena often regarded as 'processes' will be given a different interpretation in the current model, it is a mistake to believe that we can ignore all of the phonological phenomena that have been treated as processes. In particular, long-distance assimilations or dissimilations, many of which have an important role to play in development, still have to be described and monitored by the clinical phonologist. I have not investigated enough cases of harmony processes in child phonology to be able to provide an exhaustive typology. It would appear from Smith's data, for instance, that some harmony processes cannot be handled adequately in terms of simple spreading of an autosegment ('labial attraction' is just such a case). However, once the analyst has partialled out the effects of syllable and word structure constraints, and has established the child's output phoneme inventory, in many cases it will be only the assimilations which remain. As long as these can be given an informal, discursive description, this will usually be sufficient for clinical purposes.

3.2. Further implications

The model of phonological development I have presented here is more than just a way of analysing child data. It embodies a set of empirical hypotheses about what phonological development is, and should in principle be testable against empirical data. Interestingly, some of the data which might provide a particularly good test of the model should come from cases of abnormal development. Before I explain why this is so I shall describe some of the recent work of Daniel Dinnsen and his colleagues on phonological disability (see Dinnsen, Elbert, and Weismer, 1981).

I have pointed out that although we must allow for a certain degree of misperception (or at least misstorage) by normal children, the IRs are very similar to adult SRs. However, when we consider children with phonological problems it is somewhat foolhardy to make the assumption that the child has stored a correct representation of the adult form. Indeed, one might expect misperception or misstorage at this level to be a rich source of phonological impairment. I said in Chapter 5 that it is for this reason that it is somewhat puzzling that Phonological Process Analysis approaches (based on assumptions which are essentially those of the classical model) should have been so enthusiastically and uncritically taken up.

Dinnsen *et al.* point out that, if the underlying representations of a child cannot be assumed to be identical to the adult SRs, then linguistic techniques may be applied to determine what the URs actually are. A linguist confronted with this situation in analysing a new language would look for evidence from morphological alternations; that is, from the different shapes (allomorphs) which morphemes take when they undergo various processes of word formation. While English is relatively poor in morphological alternations of a kind useful in child phonology, there is one process, the formation of diminutive nouns by addition of -*i*, which provides a helpful diagnostic.

Dinnsen *et al.* distinguished a group of children in speech therapy who regularly deleted word-final consonants. Some of the children restored the deleted consonant in diminutive formation (saying, for instance, [do] for 'dog' but [dogi] for 'doggie') while others omitted the consonant even in the diminutive form (saying, for instance, [doi]). Children in the former group were said to belong to Type A, while those in the latter group belonged to Type B. The alternation evidence, together with other features of the Type A phonology, suggested that the children had intact (i.e. adult-like) URs and that the SRs reflected the operation of a rule (process) of consonant deletion. However, from a linguistic point of view there was no evidence that the Type B children had underlying final consonants in the first place. Thus, such children could not be ascribed a consonant deletion process; rather their problem was in faulty storage.

If the child's UR is his only stored form, and if Type B children store 'incorrect' URs, we would expect that these children would also have difficulty perceiving precisely those contrasts they are unable to make in their own speech. Type A children, however, who have stored the correct form, should have no such difficulty. Unfortunately the Indiana group is somewhat equivocal about this prediction. The facts of the matter seem to be that children belonging to Type B do not necessarily exhibit greater difficulty in perceptual discrimination than Type A children. This, then, is a potential source of conceptual difficulty for the theory of Dinnsen *et al.*

The current model is more highly articulated than that of Dinnsen *et al.*, who in effect adopt the simple 'two box' assumptions of the classical model. This means that the current model predicts a more varied pattern of disability than that predicted by Dinnsen *et al.* While Dinnsen *et al.* assume that input problems can manifest themselves solely at the level of IRs (in my terminology), the current model leaves open the possibility that a child's surface patterning may be the result of (a) inadequate IRs, i.e. the perceptual filter is too active; (b) inadequate URs, i.e. contrasts are lost from the OPURs because of the operation of the realisation rules; (c) inadequate SRs, despite appropriate IRs and OPURs, because of the operation of a pronunciation rule.

The effects of case (c) will be essentially those of Dinnsen *et al.*'s Type A. One would particularly look for instances in which the underlying contrast which, we assume, is still coded in the OPURs, is realised in a non-adult manner (as in the compensatory lengthening examples discussed by Dinnsen *et al.*). The effects of cases (a) and (b) subsume those of Type B. This means that the current model predicts a more finely grained typology than that of Dinnsen *et al.* In particular, it predicts that the Type B children should fall into two groups. Type B1 will have faulty IRs. Such children would be unable to perceive adequately (in linguistic contexts, at least) the contrasts they cannot make. Type B2 children, in whom the IRs are adequate but the OPURs fail to show the relevant contrasts, should behave like the Type B1 children in showing no overt sign in production of knowing the contrasts, but should be able to make those discriminations perceptually.

If research fails to uncover the two subgroups B1 and B2 then a theory along the lines of Dinnsen *et al.* will be preferable to the model presented here, and I will have to provide strong additional arguments to explain why the predicted pattern of disability does not occur. Admittedly, in fairness to the model, just because a given level of representation such as the OPURs has to be hypothesised doesn't mean automatically that a form of phonological disability affecting just that level will necesarily be observed. However, such a negative finding would certainly rouse suspicions. On the other hand, if the B1 vs. B2 distinction does prove empirically justified, this will be strong evidence in favour of the present model against all 'two box' models.

REFERENCES

Anderson, J. and Jones, C. (1974) Three theses concerning phonological representations. *Journal of Linguistics, 10*, 1-26

Anderson, S. (1985) *Phonology in the twentieth century*, University of Chicago Press, Chicago

Archangeli, D. (1984) *Underspecification in Yawelmani phonology and morphology*, MIT PhD dissertation

Cairns, C. and Feinstein, M. (1982) Markedness and the theory of syllable structure. *Linguistic Inquiry, 13*, 193-226

Chomsky, N. and Halle, M. (1968) *The sound pattern of English*, Harper & Row, New York

Clements, G. (1980) Vowel harmony in nonlinear generative phonology: an autosegmental model. Distributed by Indiana University Linguistics Club, Bloomington, Indiana

Clements, G. and Goldsmith, J. (eds) (1985) *Autosegmental studies in Bantu tone*, Foris, Dordrecht

Clements, G. and Keyser, J. (1983) *CV phonology*, MIT Press, Cambridge, Mass.

Crystal, D. (1980) *Profiling Linguistic Disability*, Edward Arnold, London

Dinnsen, D., Elbert, M. and Weismer, G. (1981) Some typological properties of functional misarticulating systems. In W.O. Dressler (ed.), *Phonologica 1980*, Innsbrucker Beitrage zur Sprachwissenschaft, Innsbruck, pp. 83-8

Edwards, M.-L. and Shriberg, L. (1983) *Phonology*, College-Hill Press, Baltimore

Fischer-Jørgensen, E. (1975) *Trends in phonological theory: a historical introduction*, Akademisk Forlag, Copenhagen

Fudge, E. (1969) Syllables. *Journal of Linguistics, 5*, 253-86

Gandour, J. (1981) The nondeviant nature of deviant phonological systems. *Journal of Communication Disorders, 14*, 11-29

Goldsmith, J. (1976) *Autosegmental phonology*. MIT PhD dissertation (published by Garland Press, New York, 1979)

Gussenhoven, C. (1983) Focus, mode and the nucleus. *Journal of Linguistics, 19*, 377-418

Halle, M. (1959) *The sound pattern of Russian*. Mouton, Den Haag

Halle, M. and Clements, G. (1983) *Problem book in phonology*, MIT Press, Cambridge, Mass.

Hawkins, P. (1982) *Phonology*, Hutchinson, London

Hooper, J. (1972) The syllable in phonological theory. *Language, 48*, 525-40

Hooper, J. (1976) *Introduction to natural generative phonology*, Academic Press, New York

Hulst, H. van der and Smith, N. (1982) An overview of Autosegmental and Metrical Phonology. In H. van der Hulst and N. Smith (eds), *The structure of phonological representations*, Part I, Foris, Dordrecht

Hulst, H. van der and Smith N. (1984) The framework of nonlinear generative phonology. In H. van der Hulst and N. Smith (eds), *Advances in nonlinear phonology*, Foris, Dordrecht

Hyman, L. (1975) *Phonology: theory and analysis*, Holt, Rinehart & Winston, New York

Ingram, D. (1976) *Phonological disability in children*, Arnold, London

Kahn, D. (1976) Syllable-based generalisations in English phonology, MIT, PhD dissertation (published by Garland Press, New York, 1980)

Kenstowicz, M. and Kisseberth, C. (1979) *Generative phonology*,

Academic Press, London

Kiparsky, P. (1982) From cyclic phonology to Lexical Phonology. In H. van der Hulst and N. Smith (eds), *The structure of phonological representations*, Part I, Foris, Dordrecht

Kiparsky, P. (1985) Some consequences of Lexical Phonology. *Phonology Yearbook, 2*, 83-136

Liberman, M. (1975) The intonational system of English. MIT PhD dissertation (published by Garland Press, New York, 1980)

Liberman, M. and Pierrehumbert, J. (1984) Intonational invariance under changes in pitch range and length. In M. Aronoff and R. Oehrle, (eds), *Language Sound Structure*, MIT Press, Cambridge, Mass.

Liberman, M. and Prince, A. (1977) On stress and linguistic rhythm. *Linguistic Inquiry, 8*, 249-336

McCarthy, J. (1979) Formal problems in Semitic phonology and morphology. MIT PhD dissertation (distributed by Indiana University Linguistics Club, Bloomington, 1982)

McCarthy, J. (1981) A prosodic theory of nonconcatenative morphology. *Linguistic Inquiry, 12*, 373-418

Macken, M. (1980) The child's lexical representation: the puzzle–puddle–pickle evidence. *Journal of Linguistics, 16*, 1-17

Schane, S. (1973) *Generative phonology*, Prentice-Hall, Englewood Cliffs, N.J.

Smith, N.V. (1973) *The acquisition of phonology*, Cambridge University Press, Cambridge

Sommerstein, A. (1977) *Phonological theory*, Arnold, London

Spencer, A. (1984) A nonlinear analysis of phonological disability. *Journal of Communication Disorders, 17*, 325-48

Spencer, A. (1986) Towards a theory of phonological development. *Lingua, 68*, 3-38

Stampe, D. (1979) *A dissertation on natural phonology*, Garland Press, New York

Stanley, R. (1967) Redundancy rules in phonology. *Language, 43*, 393-436

Venneman, T. (1972) On the theory of syllabic phonology. *Linguistische Berichte, 18*, 1-18

7

Apraxia of Speech: the Case for a Cognitive Phonetics

Chris Code and Martin J. Ball

A central issue for many years in clinical linguistics has been the question of the status of apraxia of speech. Essentially, argument has centred on whether apraxia of speech is best seen in terms of impairment of linguistic (phonological) or phonetic components of the standard generative model of the grammar. Research has attempted to describe and explain the phenomenon as arising through neurological impairments at either an abstract and more conceptual level or a concrete–motor level. However, application of the standard linguistic model to the problem appears to have reached the stage where it is unable to resolve the question of the nature of apraxia of speech. In what follows we ask why this is so and consider alternative approaches which may hold more promise for an improvement in our understanding.

A critical examination of the research completed in recent years shows that linguistic description on its own is unable to differentiate between apraxia of speech and aphasia. Linguistics, if taken to exclude all apsects of phonetics, cannot account for the phenomenon of apraxia of speech, and conversely, phonetics, if taken to exclude all aspects of linguistics, does not accomplish this task either.

We start by considering some fundamental misconceptions about the nature of apraxia of speech. These misconceptions arise because of a tendency to take too narrow a view of the interpretation of evidence from empirical research. Apraxia of speech is not an isolated impairment that can be explained *either* as a phonological *or* or a phonetic disorder just because those are components of the standard model of the grammar. Indeed, the clinical evidence shows that apraxia can affect various aspects, perhaps all aspects, of human action.

152

THE NATURE OF APRAXIA

Traditionally, a variety of forms of apraxia have been described, including ideational, ideomotor, constructional and limb-kinetic (Liepmann, 1900; Geshwind, 1975; Hecaen and Albert, 1978; Miller, 1986); although the taxonomy has undergone much criticism over the years, and there have been recent attempts to clarify the position using information-processing approaches (Roy, 1978, 1982). Even so, apraxia is understood as an impairment in the planning, initiating and co-ordinating of an action or action sequence, at the cognitive level. In contrast, an holistically produced automatic action, under closed-loop control, does not involve sequentially executed stages.

Apraxia is a definite phenomenon — it exists. There are patients who present with the disorder. Apraxia of speech (since the time of Hughlings Jackson and Liepmann) has been seen as limb-kinetic apraxia. This is classically defined as some impairment in the ability to perform purposeful, voluntary movements in the absence of neuromuscular disorder. The individual's ability to perform involuntary or automatic actions is relatively preserved. Thus a patient with a buccofacial–oral apraxia may be unable to lick his/her lips to command and even to imitation, but will automatically lick the lips while drinking a cup of tea. The implication is that voluntary and involuntary neurophysiological control over the same movement patterns, carried out by the same muscle groups, are inititated and/or organised separately. The problem with apraxia of speech is to fit this phenomenon into the traditional model of speech production having a central abstract–conceptual level mapping onto a peripheral concrete–motor level (see Figure 7.1).

Figure 7.1: The standard model

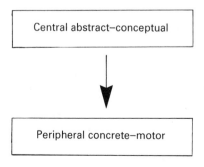

Typically, patients with apraxia of speech are said to 'know what they want to say', but are simply unable to access the required phonoarticulatory motor programmes to express the utterance. The evidence shows that patients 'know' the lexical item required and are able to demonstrate that they know it in comprehension tasks, and are able to express the meaning through non-verbal modes of expression. Examined more closely, this explanation is a 'motor explanation': the problem for the patient lies at a level of information processing somewhere between the central abstract–conceptual and peripheral concrete–motor levels. This stage is illustrated as a broad cognitive and more specific linguistic level in Figure 7.2, together with the type of impairment we suggest results from compromises of any processing stage.

Figure 7.2: The proposed model

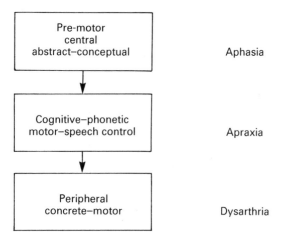

The problem then does not lie with the phonoarticulatory mechanisms themselves (witness the patient's ability to perform the same action sequence *when it is automatic*), but at the *cognitive* level. Here the problem is actually at the more abstract representational level, where 'planning' and 'co-ordination' are encoded. We return to this notion, and its implications for a model of the grammar, in more detail later.

THE LINGUISTIC STATUS OF APRAXIA OF SPEECH

If we examine the studies which have conducted linguistic and/ or phonetic investigations of apraxia of speech, we can conclude that the findings of many of these studies have more to do with the type of analysis (i.e. 'linguistic' or 'phonetic') employed. That is to say, it appears that linguistic analyses find phenomena which are describable in linguistic terms, whereas instrumental phonetic studies have found phenomena which are interpreted as being due to motor impairment. Should we put more credence on the 'harder' instrumental evidence, and conclude that apraxia of speech is a motor impairment? Or is it the case that the question of the status of apraxia of speech (linguistic vs phonetic) is not directly answerable by application of the current standard model of the grammar?

A speech disorder by definition has phonological implications, and is therefore describable as part of linguistics. That is to say, producing an error like 'b' in the initial position of the word *pan* instead of /p/ has linguistic implications, but it does not imply that the underlying cause of the error is linguistic. Such an error could be produced by dysarthria, for example, where the speech errors are due to impairment in muscular tone or co-ordination.

The problem, for linguistic interpretation, is whether the 'b' produced in the error above should be characterised as /b/ or [b] (i.e. as phonemic or phonetic). This means that simply perceiving the error does not allow us to answer the /b/ or [b] question. If a dysarthric speaker produces such an error, the cause is motoric and not linguistic. Although the error may have linguistic implications, in the sense that listeners may hear the word *ban* rather than the intended *pan*, the problem is not due to impaired *linguistic* processing. In contrast, the aphasic patient who produces the same error, and is free from dysarthria, is said to have a linguistic disorder at the syntagmatic or selectional level of competence. There is no neuromuscular reason *why* the error should have occurred. Where, then, does apraxia of speech fit in? We clearly need to look at a stage of processing intermediate between the traditional phonological and phonetic components; a stage which transforms thought into action; phonological specifications into phonetic realisation. We can identify this stage as a *phonetic programming* stage.

155

The case for considering apraxia of speech as a disorder of phonetic programming gains support from a range of sources. A respect for the experimental evidence demands that we recognise that sophisticated and complex programming levels exist between abstract central processes and peripheral motor phonetic levels (see Figure 7.2). It is here that we need to look to account for apraxia of speech.

To summarise thus far, two different levels of breakdown have traditionally been described in apraxia of speech: the more concrete–motor level (the phonetic level) or the more abstract conceptual level (the phonological level). What we have suggested is the need to examine a third alternative: an intermediate phonetic programming level.

STUDIES OF APRAXIA OF SPEECH

In terms of surface output apraxia of speech can be described as disordered phonology and, at the segmental level at least, the error types produced by the fluent aphasic and the non-fluent aphasic patient do not differ significantly. However, some linguistic analyses have suggested that because the errors produced by many apraxic patients are phonologically describable, then the underlying 'fault' is in the phonological component of the grammar. Thus a cluster reduction process (e.g. /pl/ → [p]), a deletion of marked member process (e.g. /str/ → [st]), and a manipulation of marked member process (e.g. /sl/ → [st]) characterise the great majority of errors observed in cluster production in apraxic speakers (examples from Johns and Darley, 1970; Crary and Fokes, 1980). However, the *phonetic* strategy which underlies them all is articulatory simplification. In other words, the substitution is invariably motorically easier than the target. On a linguistic interpretation of markedness no aphasic group (including those with apraxia of speech) has 'articulatory' difficulty. A contemporary appreciation, however (MacNeilage, 1982), makes it clear that markedness reflects *articulatory* properties and not linguistic ones. The patient makes *phonetic decisions* entailing cognitive planning.

A number of instrumental studies have produced evidence to support the position that apraxia of speech is a 'motor' disorder (Blumstein, Cooper, Goodglass, Statlender and Gottlieb, 1980; Blumstein, Cooper, Zurif and Caramazza, 1977; Code and Ball,

1982; Freeman, Sands and Harris, 1978; Harmes, Daniloff, Hoffman, Lewis, Kramer and Absher, 1984; Itoh, Sasanuma, Hirose, Yoshioka and Ushijima, 1980; Itoh, Sasanuma and Ushijima, 1979; Shankweiler and Harris, 1966; Johns and Darley, 1970; Johns and LaPointe, 1976. We would like to illustrate this by describing one instrumental analysis in more detail. This single case study (Code and Ball, 1982) has been replicated by another group of independent researchers with a larger group of subjects (Harmes *et al.*, 1984). The fricative production of a patient classified on standard criteria as a non-fluent 'Broca's' aphasic with apraxia of speech and no sign of dysarthria, was subjected to spectrographic analysis. The patient presented with a mild articulatory impairment which appeared only to affect friction. The most noticeable feature was a consistent devoicing of all fricatives: the patient was unable to produce voiced fricatives either in words or in isolation. It was reasoned that if the impairment were due to an underlying phonetic disfunction, then the patient would attempt to achieve phonemic contrast in his or her speech through manipulation of the phonetic features which signal lenis fricatives in English. The three primary features which distinguish a lenis (or 'voiced') from a fortis (or 'voice-less') English fricative are (a) presence (vs absence) or vocal fold vibration to varying degrees dependent on the position of the fricative in the word; (b) duration of the friction (lenis fricatives have shorter friction than fortis); and (c) preceding vowel duration (vowels before lenis fricatives are longer than those before fortis) (Grimson, 1962).

The results of the study showed (a) the subject had a selective inability to produce vocal fold vibration in voiced lenis fricatives; (b) preceding vowel durations for lenis and fortis target fricatives were normal when compared with normative data. However, the subject produced longer friction duration for both lenis and fortis target fricatives than normal subjects, and while differences between friction duration were in the same direction as in normal subjects, these differences were less. However, the subject was obviously attempting to maintain the friction duration parameter. Our results suggested that the subject was able to manipulate two of the three features necessary to make a phonological distinction between fortis and lenis fricatives, and that the impairment was not at the phonological level. If the patient's problems were due to an impaired phonology then a straightforward phonemic substitution would have taken place (e.g. /v/ would have been substituted for /f/), and no durational differences would have been observed. Moreover, the preceding vowel duration feature was also preserved, indicating a normally functioning phonology. The patient apparently had a selective impairment in the ability to initiate vocal fold vibration for fricatives.

FLUENCY

Phonetic and phonological study has been unable to distinguish, at a segmental level, between fluent aphasia and apraxia of speech. It is in fact the suprasegmental dimension of *fluency* which appears to be the most important means of distinguishing between aphasic and apraxia production errors.

A range of studies have shown that impairments of a variety of suprasegmental aspects of speech — for example, melodic line, rate of utterance, phrase length, articulatory agility — produce the typical hesitant 'stuttering-like' speech, articulatory searching and 'groping' and agrammatic speech of the Broca's motor aphasic (Kerschensteiner, Poeck and Brunnen, 1972). The speech of the typical Broca's patient with anterior left hemisphere damage is characterised by non-fluency, whereas the typical Wernicke's patient is fluent, often to the extent that speech is characterised by a verbose and logoreic jargonaphasia. The speech production of the Broca's and Wernicke's patient can be distinguished on the basis of presence or absence of disturbed fluency (Buckingham, 1979).

Apraxia of speech is a phenomenon in the world and it is the dimension of fluency that we use to distinguish between apraxia of speech and aphasia. We have seen that the standard model of the grammar is unable to capture this essential fact.

IMPLICATIONS FOR MODELS OF THE GRAMMAR: THE NEED FOR A COGNITIVE PHONETICS COMPONENT

The preceding discussion has suggested that the traditional characterisation of the relationship between phonology and phonetics is unable to account for apraxia of speech in a satisfactory way. Indeed, it is certain suprasegmental and *extralin-*

158

guistic features that appear to characterise apraxia of speech. So, is there a role for core linguistics to play in the search for understanding?

Hewlett (1985) also notes that phonetics and phonology have usually been kept apart, with phonology a branch of linguistics, whereas phonetics is not so considered. This strict separation only allows apraxia of speech to be explained as being due to damage to either component. This is not helpful for our attempt to account for the effects of apraxia of speech, as we have seen, and it is interesting therefore to note other recent suggestions to abandon the conventional division.

A recent strong advocate of this approach is Bailey (1985). Writing from the standpoint of phonetic transcription, rather than clinical linguistics, Bailey states that both phonetics and phonology should be considered parts of an overall, 'umbrella', discipline he terms 'phonetology'. He says that '*Phonetology* is a cover term that embraces both phonetics and phonology; it implies that the two disciplines, though distinct, cannot be profitably or reasonably investigated apart from each other' (Bailey, 1985, p. xii).

The notion of an overall term to cover all aspects of speech, both speech sounds and their organisation in language, is indeed appealing, and this coinage is arguably long overdue. However, Bailey does not go into details on the precise nature of the components he envisages as part of phonetology. It seems likely that three levels of unit can be used in his framework. Phones and phonemes appear in his work in their usual bracketings (square and slant respectively), but the term 'phoneteme' is also used. This is defined by Bailey as follows: 'The underlying segment, appearing between double slashes (// //), is the *phoneteme*, which is not confined to particular idiolects or styles ..., but is polylectal' (Bailey, 1985, p. xii). Earlier, Bailey had noted that his approach attempted to account for language variation, and this definition of the phoneteme reflects this. This three-level approach clearly adds a higher level of abstraction, enabling the researcher to establish a set of underlying sound units common to all lects of a language, with phoneme systems differing from lect to lect. Bailey does not make it clear, however, what the status of these phonetemes is. Are they simply artefacts enabling the phonologist to produce economical statements, or are they somehow reflecting speakers'

159

intuitions? This is not the place to review the evidence as to whether speakers of different (often markedly different) accents all have the same internalised phonetological system, but clearly this is a question that must be addressed if phonetological theory is to advance beyond the purely transcriptional.

As yet, then, Bailey's proposals do not constitute a theory coherent enough to deal with the problem outlined above. What is interesting, however, is to see the emergence of a three-tier model. In the remainder of this account we intend to examine two other proposals for three-level models of speech, the evidence for which is drawn from both normal and disordered speech.

The first of these is Hewlett's (1985). Hewlett's aim was to try to clear up some of the confusions in the use of the terms 'phonetic' and 'phonological' as applied to speech disorders. Evidence for this can be found in Hawkins (1985) who, in his summing up of the usage of the terms 'phonetic' and 'phonological', notes that speakers often comprehend distinctions they cannot make, and may attempt to produce a distinction that is not successfully conveyed to the listener. These comments suggest a complexity not adequately accounted for in a binary classification. Hawkins's comments were made on a previous contribution to this discussion by Harris and Cottam (1985). They also encounter this problem, and in their conclusion on one case study, state: 'Our supposition then is that the adult [+continuant] versus [−continuant] contrast is present in Mike's "underlying" phonological system and that its phonetic manifestation is disrupted by the intervention of lower-level articulatory processes, specifically those associated with articulatory weakening' (Harris and Cottam, 1985, p. 73).

Should this be classed as a phonological problem, as the surface realisation of Mike's problem may often be manifested as 'phoneme substitution', or phonetic as, following the quotation, other evidence suggests that the underlying phonological contrast is being maintained? This echoes the dilemma of the Code and Ball (1982) study described above.

Grunwell (1985), in a contribution to the same forum debate, notes that the difference between descriptive and explanatory accounts must be remembered: the former being data-oriented, the latter speaker-oriented. The investigation of apraxia of speech would seem to call for a speaker-oriented approach as being the more insightful. Indeed, as we noted above in the case of Bailey's work, a simple descriptive approach is limited in its application. We have also discussed the problem of separating apraxia from aphasia (for example) in a data-oriented approach.

Hewlett's proposals to overcome some of the difficulties noted by Hawkins, and Harris and Cottam, involve the positing of a three-level model of speech control. In introducing this he describes three different types of speech error. Adopting a speaker-oriented approach he offers an analysis of errors 'in terms of the process by which the error was created' (Hewlett, 1985, p. 158). The first type concerned a speaker choosing to utter a sound unit other than that of the target utterance; the second involves the choice of the correct sound unit by the speaker, but the actual realisation is slightly distorted as compared with the target sound. The third type again involves the speaker choosing the correct unit, but the phonetic production involves greater distortion such that the resultant sound is identical (or virtually so) to another phonemic unit.

Hewlett's example involves attempts at a target /s/. The first error type can be illustrated by the speaker choosing to produce the phonological unit /t/ instead of /s/, and uttering [t]. The second type of error involves the choice of /s/, but the slight distortion of this in production to [ʂ]. The third type again involves the choice of /s/, but the greater distortion produces a phonetic realisation of [t].

Hewlett recognises the difficulties in attempting this distinction, based on a concept of speaker's phonological choice that is not directly observable. The surface realisations of type one and type three above are, in this example, of course identical, though the motivations are not. Hewlett suggests that significant insights may be gained by considering *patterns* of phonetic realisations rather than just individual instances. In a similar example, Harris and Cottam (1985) comment on Mike's use of the [continuant] feature. They note, 'this conclusion [i.e. that the contrast exists at an underlying level] is partially supported by his high success rate in auditory discrimination tests based on this distinction' (p. 73). Hawkins (1985) also notes discrimination tests together with variability in production, as ways of investigating this aspect.

Hewlett terms speech errors 'phonological', 'phonetic' or 'articulatory'. Phonological disorders (Hewlett's first type in the example above) would be those 'involving the phonological

161

representation of words in the speaker's brain, or the mental processes used in the conversion of phonological forms into phonetic forms' (Hewlett, 1985, p. 160). At the other end of the scale, articulatory disorders are reserved for 'pathologies in which the anatomy of the vocal tract is affected' (p. 162). Phonetic disorders are those where the correct phonological input is outputted incorrectly, although there are no anatomical deficiencies. Hewlett also refers to these disorders as impairments of the 'learned skills of phonetic implementation' (p. 161).

Hewlett uses examples from various pathologies to illustrate his argument for a three-level model. Of specific interest to us here are his comments on apraxia of speech. He notes that it 'provides good evidence that selecting the right phonological category and having an unimpaired vocal tract are not sufficient for the achievement of normal speech' (p. 161). He briefly discusses the need for a 'phonetic encoding' component, and his discussion of this in relation to normal speech (the fact that one must learn precisely how to encode phonological features in a language-specific way) ties in well to Tatham (1984) discussed below. Hewlett extends his argument to the area of phonological disorders in children. He argues that in many cases the examination of comprehension suggests that children have the correct phonological form of words stored mentally but simply are unable to produce them (e.g. 'not wabbit, *wabbit*'). Again, this suggests an impairment at a level of phonetic encoding rather than execution, as often the sounds in question can be produced in isolation or as imitation.

Hewlett associates his three-level model with the work of Mlcoch and Noll (1980), which has subsequently appeared in revised form in Mlcoch and Square (1984). These authors present a six-component neurolinguistic model of speech production, though only four of these components are of immediate interest to us. Their *auditory speech processor* is equivalent to a phonological component, and their *primary motor area* is equivalent to a traditional articulatory phonetics component. Intermediate between these two are two encoding components: the *articulatory coder* (AC) and the *motor speech programmer* (MSP). The main difference between these two appears to be the ability to receive tactile and proprioceptive feedback.

Although this model differs from Hewlett's suggestions (and Tatham's, see below), it is interesting to note that in their discussion of the location of the impairment involved with apraxia of speech, Mlcoch and Square (1984) note that evidence suggests that the AC and/or MSP may be involved. They argue that this evidence supports the view that in apraxia the feedback role of the AC may be affected, as several investigations indicate that oral sensory perceptual deficits occur frequently among apraxic speakers (see Deutsch, 1984, for review). Other apraxic errors, however, suggest impairment at the level of the MSP. These include errors involving initiating, transitionalising, mistiming, sequencing, inco-ordination and anticipation.

If we turn back now to a somewhat more abstract linguistic approach that parallels the views of Hewlett (1985), we can conclude our discussion by looking at the work of Tatham (1984). Judging from references, it would appear that Hewlett and Tatham have come to very similar conclusions independently: Hewlett from examining disordered language, while Tatham's approach is normative.

Tatham (1984), based on original work by both Tatham and Morton (cited in Tatham, 1984), proposes the need for a 'cognitive phonetic' component, intermediate between the traditional phonological and phonetic components. Tatham argues that evidence for the existence of such a component can be found by examining the requirements of *repeatability* of the sounds of languages: that is the fact that language requires its sounds to be 'the same' each time they are used, to facilitate encoding and decoding of messages. This requirement of repeatability sets up a tension in the system, in that it may not at all times and in all contexts be necessary for the articulatory configuration of a particular sound to be identical. In other words, the immediate context may provide cues to a hearer, such that the articulatory constraints on a sound can be relaxed without the possibility of confusion resulting. As Tatham (1984) notes, 'Such a system is an active one which actually "considers" whether context might alter one-to-one object-encoding (and decoding) to enable some improvement in the system's efficiency' (p. 41).

This notion of relaxation of articulatory constraints is termed 'articulatory wobble' by Tatham (1984), who goes on to discuss in detail the advantages and disadvantages of this feature, together with a discussion of some of the factors affecting it (for example, high ambient noise may well stop the relaxation of articulatory constraints).

163

A final example from Tatham's work echoes some of the ideas of Hewlett (1985). This concerns cross-language comparisons of phonetic precision. Tatham notes that the precision required to separate /s/ from /ʃ/ in English is absent in Spanish, which has only one fricative phoneme in this articulatory domain. Tatham notes that 'this Spanish fricative has a relatively large domain with less linguistic constraint on wobble' (p. 44). A similar example concerns VOT in languages with a two-way VOT contrast system (as English), as compared to those with a three-way contrast system (as Hindi or Korean). The allowable amount of wobble in the realisation of the VOT contrasts is greater in the two-way system.

These examples clearly fit in with Hewlett's (1985) statement that 'the way in which a similar phonological distinction is realised phonetically in two different languages is always slightly different' (p. 161). Indeed, both authors refer to this intermediate component as a phonetic encoder: 'cognitive phonetics is therefore about the mental processes involved during the encoding and decoding of the final stages of transforming thought into sound'. Tatham continues:

> it is about what has to be considered when inputting an idealized phonological requirement with a view to outputting a soundwave which has to be decoded back to some copy, as little degraded as necessary, of the original thought. It is about considering the manipulation or recruitment of implementing mechanisms, on a long-term, short-term or on-going basis. It is about *mental control* of the control of those mechanisms (Tatham, 1984, p. 46).

Tatham, then, is proposing a new component, part of linguistics, but separate from phonology. He concludes that cognitive phonetics is proposed to take the role previously assigned to a non-abstract phonetics in its relationship to phonology. 'It is the component of the grammar following the phonology, and it is responsible for what in phonology is phonetically determined' (p. 47).

CONCLUSION

What we have been discussing here is a three-level 'phonetology' (to use Bailey's term), straddling the traditional linguistics–

phonetics divide. This phonetology consists of a phonological component, containing the abstract, mental, phonemic representations of words. Next we have the cognitive phonetic component which is concerned, in an active way, with phonetic encoding. Finally, there is an articulatory phonetic component, responsible for realising the motor stage of speech production.

Using this model we can refer back to the speaker-oriented taxonomy of speech and language disorders in terms of their linguistic location (see Figure 7.2). In particular for our purposes we can examine its use with impairments in adult-acquired disorders. An impairment of the articulatory phonetic component is illustrated in dysarthria, whereas impairment at the cognitive phonetic component is seen in apraxia of speech, and an impairment at the phonological level may be found in aphasia.

Naturally, refinements of such a model are expected, particularly in the light of Mlcoch and Noll's work. Cognitive phonetics cannot actually help distinguish apraxic from dysarthric from aphasic speech. That requires a data-oriented approach as taken by those studies which have employed the fluency dimension. However, the notion of a cognitive phonetic level as being the location of the disfunction in apraxia of speech is one we feel to be of longstanding importance.

REFERENCES

Bailey, C.-J.N. (1985) *English phonetic transcription*, University of Texas, and Summer Institute of Linguistics, Arlington

Blumstein, S., Cooper, W.E., Goodglass, H., Statlender, S. and Gottlieb, J. (1980) Production deficits in aphasia: a voice-onset-time analysis. *Brain and Language*, 9, 153-70

Blumstein, S., Cooper, W.E., Zurif, E.B. and Caramazza, A. (1977) The perception and production of voice onset time in aphasia. *Neuropsychologia*, 15, 371-83

Buckingham, H. (1979) Explanation in apraxia with consequences for the concept of apraxia of speech. *Brain and Language*, 8, 202-26

Code, C. (1984) Delayed auditory feedback. In C. Code and M. Ball (eds), *Experimental clinical phonetics*. Croom Helm, London

Code, C. and Ball, M.J. (1982) Fricative production in Broca's aphasia: a spectrographic analysis. *Journal of Phonetics*, 10, 325-31

Crary, M. and Fokes, J. (1980) Phonological processes in apraxia of speech: a systematic simplification of articulatory performance. *Aphasia Apraxia Agnosia*, 4, 1-13

Deutsch, S.E. (1984) Oral stereognosis. In C. Code and M.J. Ball (eds),

Experimental Clinical Phonetics. Croom Helm, London

Freeman, F.J., Sands, E.S. and Harris, K.S. (1978) Temporal coordination of phonation and articulation in a case of verbal apraxia: a voice onset time study. *Brain and Language*, *6*, 106-11

Geschwind, N. (1975) The apraxias: neural mechanisms of disorders of learned movement. *American Scientist*, *63*, 188-95

Gimson, A.C. (1962) *An introduction to the pronunciation of English*. Edward Arnold, London

Grunwell, P. (1985) Comment on the terms 'phonetics' and 'phonology' as applied in the investigation of speech disorders. *British Journal of Disorders of Communication*, *20*, 165-70

Harmes, S., Daniloff, R., Hoffman, P., Lewis, J., Kramer, M. and Absher, R. (1984) Temporal and articulatory control of fricative articulation by speakers with Broca's aphasia. *Journal of Phonetics*, *12*, 367-85

Harris, J. and Cottam, P. (1985) Phonetic features and phonological features in speech assessment. *British Journal of Disorders of Communication*, *20*, 61-74

Hawkins, P. (1985) A tutorial comment on Harris and Cottam. *British Journal of Disorders of Communication*, *20*, 75-80

Hecaen, H. and Albert, M.L. (1978) *Human neuropsychology*, Wiley, New York

Hewlett, N. (1985) Phonological versus phonetic disorders: some suggested modifications to the current use of the distinction. *British Journal of Disorders of Communication*, *20*, 155-64

House, A.S. and Fairbanks, G. (1953) The influence of consonant environment upon the secondary acoustical characteristics of vowels. *Journal of the Acoustical Society of America*, *23*, 105-13

Itoh, M., Sasanuma, S., Hirose, H., Yoshioka, H. and Ushijima, T. (1980) Abnormal articulatory dynamics in a patient with apraxia of speech: x-ray microbeam observation. *Brain and Language*, *11*, 66-75

Itoh, M., Sasanuma, S. and Ushijima, T. (1979) Velar movements during speech in a patient with apraxia of speech. *Brain and Language*, *7*, 227-39

Johns, D.F. and Darley, F.L. (1970) Phonemic variability in apraxia of speech. *Journal of Speech and Hearing Research*, *13*, 556-83

Johns, D.F. and LaPointe, L.L. (1976) Neurogenic disorders of output processing: apraxia of speech. In H. Whitaker and H.A. Whitaker (eds), *Studies in neurolinguistics*, vol. 1, Academic Press, New York

Kerschensteiner, M., Poeck, K. and Brunnen, E. (1972) The fluency–non-fluency dimension in the classification of aphasic speech. *Cortex*, *8*, 233-47

Liepmann, H. (1900) Das Krankheitsbild der Apraxie (motorischen Asymbolie) auf Grund eines Falles von einseitiger Apraxie. *Monatschrift fuer Psychiatrie und Neurologie*, *8*, 15-40, 102-32, 182-97

MacNeilage, P.F. (1982) Speech production mechanisms in aphasia. In S. Grillner, B. Lindblom, J. Lubker and A. Perrson, (eds), *Speech motor control*, Pergamon Press, Oxford

Miller, N. (1986) *Dyspraxia and its Management*, Croom Helm,

London

Mlcoch, A. and Noll, J. (1980) Speech production models as related to the concept of apraxia of speech. In N.J. Lass (ed.), *Speech and language: advances in basic research and practice*, vol. 4, Academic Press, New York

Mlcoch, A. and Square, P. (1984) Apraxia of speech: articulatory and perceptual factors. In N.J. Lass (ed.), *Speech and language: advances in basic research and practice*, vol. 10, Academic Press, New York

Peterson, G.E. and Lehiste, I. (1960) Duration of syllable nuclei in English. *Journal of the Acoustical Society of America*, *32*, 693-703

Roy, E.A. (1978) Apraxia: a new look at an old syndrome. *Journal of Human Movement Studies*, *4*, 191-210

Roy, E.A. (1982) Action and performance. In A.W. Ellis (ed.), *Normality and pathology in cognitive functions*, Academic Press, London

Shankweiler, D. and Harris, K.S. (1966) An experimental approach to the problem of articulation in aphasia. *Cortex*, *11*, 277-92

Tatham, M.A.A. (1984) Towards a *cognitive* phonetics. *Journal of Phonetics*, *12*, 37-47

8

The Contribution of Speech Pathology to the Development of Phonetic Description

Martin J. Ball

INTRODUCTION

In his recent important contribution to the development of phonetic transcription, Bailey (1985) notes, 'It is regrettable that at a time when phonetic research has been making great strides forward, phonetic transcription methods have been moving backwards' (p. ix). A similar feeling was expressed by Canepari (1983): 'This work has grown from a well-known sense of uneasiness that accompanies most phoneticians ... that is due to various factors: first, the lack of an adequate number of signs to transcribe particular sounds' (p. 19). Canepari also notes the problems of differing phonetic transcription traditions, and degrees of phonetic training.

These two authors are expressing dissatisfaction with current practices in impressionistic phonetic transcription. That is to say, with that area of phonetic description which uses a symbol system to record the phonetician's auditory perceptions. The most widely used of these symbol systems is the International Phonetic Alphabet (IPA, PIPA 1949, and 1979). Both the works cited are attempts at expanding this alphabet, and applying it more rigorously, though Bailey is mostly concerned with English transcription.

Impressionistic transcription is, however, only one arm of phonetic description. Over the past 40 years or so, instrumental phonetics has made great advances, so that we now have many techniques available to aid us in phonetic descriptions of both articulatory and acoustic features of speech. Instrumental phonetics also gives the investigator a permanent record, not in the form of written symbols, but usually, in the first place, in the form of electrical signals. These electrical signals can be converted into more manageable records. As Tatham (1984) notes:

> In work in speech we generally make two kinds of record: (1) a recording of the actual data, obtained as closely as possible to the original conversion of the information into electrical signals, and (2) a visual recording of the final output of any electrical or other processing of the data for the inspection and measuring by the investigator (p. 1).

Tatham goes on to point out that method (1) generally involves tape-recording, whereas (2) usually means chart recording on paper.

Impressionistic transcription and instrumental transcription are, then, the two branches of phonetic description, cutting across subdivisions of phonetics in terms of subject-matter (i.e. articulatory, acoustic or auditory phonetics). As noted in the references cited above, concern over the efficacy of impressionistic transcription is being voiced increasingly by phoneticians, whereas instrumental (or 'experimental') phonetics has been expanding, and its appeal as a way of surmounting problems in phonetic description, increasing.

However, in practical terms impressionistic transcription still has many advantages over an instrumental approach. Anyone trained in the use of the IPA (or similar symbol system) can undertake a transcription quickly (sometimes even simultaneous with the utterance(s)). This means it is immediately available for examination and analysis. Also, it is available for examination by other phoneticians trained in that symbol system. Instrumental phonetics, on the other hand, is rarely so accessible. Firstly, the instruments themselves (often costly) need to be acquired, and phoneticians trained in their use. Analysis via the machines can be somewhat time-consuming (though rarely excessively so), and the end results need to be interpreted. Learning how to undertake the interpretation is not always a straightforward matter, comparable to some extent to learning a symbol system. Finally, replication of analyses is only open to phoneticians with the same instruments, as is — in many cases — analysis of the permanent records. On a practical level the impressionistic transcriber needs to take only his knowledge with him to a transcription session, the instrumental transcriber needs his machine!

We need now to turn our attention to the role of phonetic description in speech pathology. The speech pathologist needs access to phonetic description in a wide range of speech and language disorders, not simply for so-called 'phonetic' disorders. The distinction between phonetic and phonological problems is not always clear, and there has been much recent debate on defining these terms[1] (see Hewlett, 1985; Grunwell, 1985; Milroy, 1985 for examples). It is not necessary here for us to enter into this debate, for whether or not the phonology is affected by a speech disorder is irrelevant to the need for an accurate and comprehensive description of the sound produced. The question that arises is, should this description be impressionistic or instrumental? This chapter will argue that for the speech pathologist both approaches are often necessary, but we will be attempting to show that refinements in both areas are required if the needs of speech pathology are to be met, and to examine some developments led by speech pathology.

The disadvantages of the instrumental approach noted above apply also to the speech pathologist. For reasons of cost, many of the more useful experimental phonetic techniques may not be available; or they may not be portable to the desired place of use. On the other hand, phonetic symbolisation, as currently practised by many phoneticians, has been criticised as being inadequate for normal language, even before considering non-normal speech.

However, the increase in interest in clinical language studies has led to the development of a field of clinical phonetics, covering both the experimental side (see Code and Ball, 1984), and the impressionistic side (see PRDS, 1983). It is the purpose of this chapter to present the advances in these two areas in a comprehensive and coherent manner, and to point to the future through suggestions for further developments.

IMPRESSIONISTIC TRANSCRIPTION

Speech pathologists have long been trained in the use of impressionistic transcription, mainly through the IPA, or the slight variant of the IPA traditionally used in America. However, we need to stress at this point that impressionistic transcriptions can be used to describe different levels of abstraction. A 'narrow' or strictly phonetic transcription aims to capture in symbol form the maximum of phonetic information that the transcriber is able to perceive, and for which he has symbols. A phonemic transcription, on the other hand, includes the minimum of redundant information — precise phonetic detail being recoverable by rule. Of course, it is the strict phonetic transcription which provides the data for constructing the rules whereby phonemic transcriptions can be read: these latter being principled abstractions from information provided by the former.

Naturally, phoneticians often require a transcription whose detail is somewhere between the narrowest phonetic and the broadest phonemic approach. This can be seen, for example, in instances where narrow phonetic detail is recorded for consonants (or a particular class of consonants), but the vowels are recorded in a broad, phonemic, manner.

The use of a phonemic transcription (that is one between slant brackets, / /), does imply that some kind of analysis of the phonetic facts has taken place, and the lect being transcribed has a reasonably wide currency, or at least has been subject to previous analysis.

All these points are relevant to the problem of using impressionistic transcription in speech pathology. By definition, a patient presenting with a speech problem cannot be using (or using acceptably) a previously analysed phonemic system. Therefore, a strictly phonemic transcription of his/her speech is not going to be possible, or if attempted will be misleading. Carney (1979) pointed to this problem for the speech pathologist: 'There are however inherent dangers in using phonetic data which have been over-cooked by abstraction' (p. 123).

Carney illustrates some of these dangers. The major problem involves 'distortions' of adult target phonemes, or 'substitutions' plus 'distortions'. If a child replaces target /k/ with [t^h], then phonemicising this as /t/ presents no problem. If however /k/ is replaced by [t̪], then using /t/ to show this will obscure what might well be important information about this change, information that might be important for treatment as well as analysis.

Another example provided by Carney involves the same phone being phonemicised differently because of the expectations provoked by the target sound. If adult /f/ is realised as [ɸ], this is likely to be phonemicised as /f/. Likewise if adult /p/ is also realised as [ɸ], it is possible that this will be symbolised as /p/. Thereby the patient's loss of contrast between /p/ –/f/ is not recorded.

Carney also notes that patients' realisations are sometimes not transcribed at all if the phone used (e.g. initial glottal stop) does not appear to be relatable to any target phoneme.

This phonemic approach to the transcription of disordered speech is probably strongest in America, because of the Bloomfieldian tradition of avoiding impressionistic transcription. However, if the speech pathologist is going to use phonetic symbolisation it is hoped that the need to avoid a phonemic approach has been shown. This is not to say that every transcription of every patient must be at the extreme 'narrow' end of the transcription spectrum. As noted above, degrees of detail are available to the phonetician, and as Carney states, 'hard-pressed therapists will clearly not bother to record more phonetic detail than experience warrants to be necessary' (p. 123). This is particularly so if previous analysis of the patient's speech output has been undertaken.

What is available to the speech pathologist seeking to undertake a detailed phonetic transcription? The symbol chart of the IPA (as revised to 1979) provides 70 major consonant symbols (about half a dozen minor consonant symbols are included in footnotes). Twenty-five vowel symbols are shown on two vowel diagrams, and a range of diacritics are also provided. These diacritics show changes in place of articulation, phonation type, nasalisation, secondary articulations and so on.

With these sets of symbols and diacritics it is claimed to be possible to provide impressionistic transcriptions of any normal language that has been discovered (how efficiently is another question). However, the speech pathologist is of course not dealing with the normal. The IPA, and other transcriptions based on normal speech, do not contain symbols for some of the sounds encountered in the speech therapy clinic. Because of this, a major attempt to expand symbolisation to cope with disordered speech was made by a group of British phoneticians and speech pathologists in recent years. This group — the Phonetic Representation of Disordered Speech group — was first convened in 1979, publishing a preliminary report after a year (PRDS, 1980), with a final report later (PRDS, 1983). Grunwell (1982) describes the new symbols in an appendix, but does not use them in that publication. Little published work uses these new symbols as yet (though see Ball, Duckworth and Munro, 1984, and Ball, in preparation for examples of their use in Welsh disordered speech).

PRDS (1980) reports that its preliminary investigations among speech pathologists revealed several areas of transcription where additional symbolisation was regarded as needed: 'lack of aspiration; nasal friction; weak, strong, silent and very short articulations; labiodental plosives; ingressive fricatives; dental friction ...; a "not sure" convention and many others' (p. 216). The 1983 revision was minor, altering a few of the suggestions, and adding some more categories. This latest version is presented in Table 8.1.

It is not necessary for us to examine in detail the various categories included in this set of additional symbols;[2] the table is sufficiently detailed to do this. However, it is worth noting that the great majority of the new symbols involve diacritics being placed on existing symbols. Furthermore, the proposals concern consonantal articulations only. I intend to discuss these two aspects below in some detail.

The IPA tradition reserves the vast majority of its diacritics (though not all) to mark secondary aspects of the articulation of a segment: such as a slightly different place of articulation than normal (retracted/advanced for example), or secondary articulation (labialisation, velarisation, etc.), or aspects of stop release (aspiration for example), or segment length.[3] Ball (in preparation) criticises the American usage of symbols such as [š] for IPA [ʃ], or [ü] for IPA [y], just because a diacritic here is being used to 'alter' a primary aspect of articulation, and in doing so somehow suggests that [š] is just a slightly different sort of [s], and so on.

The same point can be made in respect of many of the PRDS suggestions. Examining Table 8.1, we find that whereas lingua-labials get separate unit symbols ([P, B, M, þ 8, L⁴]), the labio-dentals do not — indeed the IPA (ɱ) (labiodental nasal) is provided with an alternative form plus diacritic: [m̪]. Following the example of [ɱ], surely symbols such as [p̪] and [b̪] or [p] and [þ], might have been suggested?

The remaining new place of articulation suggestions nearly all involve diacritic usage. In some instances this seems justified, for example the difference between dental and interdental is indeed only one of slight advancement. However, to use the retraction diacritic for a velar lateral, by placing the diacritic on the palatal lateral symbol, is going beyond the general usage of diacritics described above. (See below for alternative solutions for the velar lateral.)

Table 8.1: Recommended phonetic symbols for the representation of segmental aspects of disordered speech

(a) Relating mainly to place of articulation

		p̱p̱p̱	b͡bb
(1) Bilabial trills			
(2) Lingualabials	plosives, nasal	p	B, M
(tongue tip/blade to upper lip)	fricatives	ᵦ	ᵦ
	lateral		ꞁ
(3) Labiodental plosives and nasal	plosives, nasal	p̪	b̪, m̪
(ɱ is an alternative to the usual m̪)			
(4) Reverse labiodentals	plosives, nasal	p̪ˌ ȶ	b̪ˌ ʋ̰
(lower teeth to upper lip)	fricatives	+ꞁ	+ꝺ
(5) Interdentals	plosives, nasal	ꞇ	+ꝺ (or ꝺ̰ etc.)
(using existing IPA convention for advancement)			
(6) Bidentals	fricatives	ꞗ	ꞓ (or ꝺ etc.)
(lower teeth to upper teeth)	percussive	)(	
(7) Voiced palatal fricative		ꞁ̇	
(reserving j for palatal approximant)			
(8) Voiced velar lateral		ʎ̱	
(using existing IPA convention for retraction)			
(9) Pharyngeal plosives		q̱	ɢ̱
(do.)			

(b) Relating mainly to manner of articulation

(10) Segments with nasal escape:
  (i) nasal fricatives (audible turbulent nasal egressive air-flow; no oral escape)

m̥ᶠ   mᶠ   n̥ᶠ   ŋᶠ   etc.

(ii) nasalized fricatives — s̃ z̃ x̃ etc.; also ʂ̃ᶠ etc.

(iii) sounds intermediate between oral stop and nasal — t̃ d̃ p̃ etc.

Note: the nasality diacritic [~] may be freely used to denote nasal resonance or escape; it does not in itself imply nasal friction, for which the raised [ᶠ] is recommended.

(11) Lateral fricatives with sibilance — ɬʃ ... ɮ³ etc.; or ɬʃ etc.

(12) Strong/tense articulation — f̬ m̬ etc.

(13) Weak/lax/tentative articulation — f̬ ... ȶ̬

*as compared with the norm for the segment in question

(14) Reiterated articulation (as in dysfluencies and palilalia) — p͡pp etc.

(15) Alveolar slit fricatives (using existing IPA convention for retraction) — θ̠ ð̠

(16) Blade (as opposed to tip of tongue) articulation — s̻

(17) Plosive with non-audible release — p̚ b̚

(c) *Relating to vocal fold activity*

(18) Unaspirated (where explicit symbolization is desired) — p⁼ t⁼ etc.

(19) Pre-voiced; post-voiced (i.e. with voicing starting earlier/continuing later than the norm for the segment in question) — ˌz z̦ etc.

(20) Partially voiced (for segments normally voiceless; use where 'ş' etc. is not sufficiently explicit) — ˌs ș etc.

(21) Partially voiceless (for segments normally voiced; use where 'ʐ' etc. is not sufficiently explicit) — ˳z z̥

(22) Preaspirated — ʰp ʰt etc.

Table 8.1 continued

(d) Relating to air-stream mechanism

(23) Pulmonic ingressive   s̩   m̩   etc.

(24) Oral (velaric) egressive   ʇ   etc.
     ('reverse click')

(25) Zero air-stream   (f)   (m)   etc.
     (absence of air-stream mechanism, but articulation present;
     'silent articulations', 'mouthing')

     Note: this may occur simultaneously with an articulation using some   ʔ(f)   ŋ(f)
     other air-stream mechanism, for example

(e) Relating to duration, coarticulation, and pausing

(26) Excessively short   m̆   ð̆   ə̆ etc.

     Note: it is felt that confusion is unlikely to arise between this use and the customary IPA use to denote non-syllabicity; but this diacritic should *not* be used to denote mere absence of length.

(27) Prolonged   m: (or m::)   etc.
     (using existing IPA conventions)   p: (i.e. with prolonged hold/closure
                                              stage)

(28) Silence, with absence of coarticulatory effects between segments or words

           short   -   thus ʌn-də

           long   --   ʌn--də

           extra long   ---   ʌn---də

(f) Relating to secondary articulation

(29) Lip rounding   s̫
     (using existing IPA convention for labialization)

(30) Lip spreading   s̪

(g) Relating to inadequacy of data or transcriptional confidence

(31) 'Not sure'

Ring doubtful symbols or cover symbols, thus

◯	entirely unspecified articulatory segment
Ⓒ	unspecified consonant
Ⓥ	unspecified vowel
Ⓢ	unspecified stop
Ⓕ	unspecified fricative
Ⓐ	unspecified approximant
(NAS)	unspecified nasal
(AFF)	unspecified affricate
(LAT)	unspecified lateral
(PAL)	probably palatal, unspecified manner (etc.)
ɫ	probably [ɫ], but not sure (etc.)
m (ɣ)(k)	probably [ɣk], but not sure (etc.)

Note: a voiced, but otherwise unspecified, fricative may be shown as Ⓕ ; similarly, a voiceless, but otherwise unspecified, stop as Ⓢ ; and so on.

(32) Speech sound(s) masked by extraneous noise

thus   (( ))
         bɪg ((bæd wʊl))f
or   bɪg ((2 sylls))

(33) *The asterisk.* It is recommended that free use be made of asterisks (indexed, if necessary) and footnotes where it is desired to record some segment or feature for which no symbol is provided.

The manner of articulation suggestions all involve diacritics or superscripts, but most of these are within the constraints on diacritic usage I have noted. This is also the case with most of the remaining sections. The use of diacritics to denote airstream mechanisms may be criticised (though of course the IPA uses ['] to denote glottalic egressive sounds), but as these are all non-normal mechanisms, any alternatives would have been grossly uneconomical.

The final section on uncertainties is a useful addition to the speech pathologist's transcriptional armoury.

The criticism on diacritic usage is made of course from the theoretical standpoint. In actual usage a diacritic that can be applied to many symbols is obviously easier to remember than a set of new symbols. Nevertheless, there is still the danger that these articulations may come to be viewed as merely minor variations of a 'normal' sound, thus leading the transcriber into the dangers noted by Carney (1979).

Canepari (1983) attempted a major expansion of the IPA, though not for the needs of the speech pathologist. Nevertheless, some of his suggestions may eventually come to be preferred to the PRDS proposals. In particular, the velar lateral, discussed above, is provided with a symbol for voiceless and for voiced: [ʟ̥, ʟ]. Interestingly enough, the problem of symbolising the velar lateral is not recent; Ladefoged, Cochran and Disner (1977), in a paper on laterals and trills, discuss the phonetics of the sound in some detail, and note that the symbol [ɡ̫] has been used to denote the sound. As Canepari is not dealing with non-normal speech, no symbols are suggested for many of the place types in PRDS (1983), but symbols are suggested for other place types which may be useful to the speech pathologist, particularly double articulations.

The other point noted above concerned vowel articulations. Firstly, vowel 'problems' are rarely transcribed by speech pathologists, probably because they rarely occur, or are rarely very noticeable (see Grunwell, 1982, p. 214). Of course, it is also possible that they are rarely transcribed because transcribers are unsure how to do this. The PRDS group have provided no special vowel symbols, presumably because the cardinal vowel system, together with the IPA lax vowel symbols and diacritics, is assumed to be adequate for a narrow vocalic transcription; or because it is assumed that clinicians will simply use a convenient phonemic transcription.

However, if we are to avoid Carney's (1979) 'inappropriate abstractions', it may well be the case that a narrow vowel transcription is needed to explain consonantal co-articulations, even if the vowel system is not to be analysed in itself. How adequate is the cardinal vowel system for this task? Leaving aside the large number of diacritics that need to be used, and their often imprecise character (see Ball, in preparation, for discussion of this), this system has been attacked strenuously recently as being inaccurate. The traditional, 'tongue-arch' model of vowel production, as used in the cardinal vowel system, has been shown to be inadequate according to Wood (1982), who, by using X-ray and other evidence, suggests a new model which provides terms for the location of vowel articulations in four main articulatory areas (palatal, velar, upper pharyngeal and lower pharyngeal).

This approach had not yet directly affected symbolisation. Canepari (1983) does not accept all of Wood's proposals, but he does recognise that the cardinal vowel system is overly simplistic. For example, front-rounded vowels are not as front as front-unrounded ones. Conversely, back-unrounded vowels are not as back as back-rounded ones. He also feels that to avoid using excessive numbers of height and front/back diacritics, vowel symbols should be provided, where appropriate, for six degrees of height, and five degrees of front/back. His resultant system is displayed in Table 8.2, taken from Canepari (1983, p. 35). The values of these vowels are included on tape-recordings accompanying Canepari (1983).

While I am not necessarily suggesting that speech pathologists must now learn a new vowel transcription system, I feel it is important that it is stressed that vowel articulations should not always be simply phonemicised to the target system; a more precise transcription is possible, and may on occasions be important (for example when accounting for co-articulations).

This section has attempted to show how the needs of speech pathologists, and the needs of phoneticians, appear to be converging in the area of impressionistic transcription. The debate is only just beginning, but the conservatism of the phonetic transcription 'establishment' is being challenged from both within and without, new practices are being adopted, and (literally) the shape of phonetic symbolisation may be in for great change.

Table 8.2:

		⊞ LIP-ROUNDING	0 FRONT	1 FRONT-CENTRAL	2 CENTRAL	3 BACK-CENTRAL	4 BACK	
CLOSE	HIGH	+	ʉ	y	ʉ	ɯ	u	A
	SEMI-HIGH	+		ʏ	ʊ	ɤ	ʊ	B
MID	HIGH-MID	+	ø	ɵ	ɤ	o		C
	LOW-MID	+	œ	ɞ	ɵ	ɔ		D
OPEN	SEMI-LOW	+	œ	ɐ	ɒ	ɔ		E
	LOW	+				ɒ		F

		⊞ ARROTONDAMENTO	5 ANTERIORE	6 ANTEROCENTRALE	7 CENTRALE	8 POSTEROCENTRALE	9 POSTERIORE	
ACCOSTO	ALTO	−	i	ʮ	ɨ	ɯ		A
	SEMIALTO	−	ɪ	ʟ	ɪ	ɰ		B
MEDIO	MEDIOALTO	−	e	ə	ə	ɤ		C
	MEDIOBASSO	−	ɛ	ɜ	ɜ	ʌ		D
APERTO	SEMIBASSO	−	ɛ	ɐ	ɐ	ʌ	ɔ	E
	BASSO	−	æ	ʌ	a	ɑ	ɑ	F

INSTRUMENTAL TRANSCRIPTION

Impressionistic transcription is not the only area of phonetic description where the needs of speech pathology have prompted innovations or suggested adaptations.

180

Naturally enough, instrumental phonetics began as a way for phoneticians to gain more precise information than was possible previously. This information might be articulatory (see for example the very early use of X-rays in phonetic description as noted in Ball, 1984), or acoustic (especially with the development of the speech spectrograph in the 1940s–Koenig, Dunn and Lacy, 1946), or auditory/perceptive. However, certain techniques have arisen specifically to help the speech pathologist's investigations, and one of these is described in detail below. Furthermore, many other techniques have been increasingly used in the study of disordered speech, and some of the more important work will be referred to in this section. As this chapter is on phonetic *description*, this section on instrumental approaches does not examine the therapeutic aspects of any of the techniques mentioned, and areas such as the use of speech aids are deemed to lie outside the scope of both the terms 'phonetic' and 'description'.

Instrumental phonetics techniques can be divided into those primarily useful for investigating articulatory events, those more helpful in examining the acoustic signal emanating from these events, and finally those concerned with auditory aspects of phonetics. It is not possible within the confines of this chapter to go into detail on all the important techniques in these areas (see Code and Ball, 1984, for a full account), so attention will be focused on those instruments felt to be most important within speech pathology.

Numerous instrumental methods are available for examining articulatory aspects of speech. For example, various types of laryngoscope have been used to examine laryngeal activity, both in terms of phonation, and pitch (see Keller, 1971, for a description of a manual laryngoscope, and Abberton and Fourcin, 1984, for an account of electrolaryngography. The use of this latter is described in more detail below).

If we wish to examine the articulation of individual sounds, palatography may be employed. Palatography attempts to show which area(s) of the roof of the mouth are involved in the articulation of particular sounds, and may be combined with linguograms which show which part of the tongue made contact with the palate, etc., in any sound. Direct palatography involves photographing the subject's palate after the articulation of the sound in question in order to examine the patterns of disturbance of a previously applied powder coating. Indirect palatography uses a 'made-to-measure' artificial palate inserted in the subject's mouth from which to take readings from a set of electrodes incorporated into this device. The methods are fully described in Keller (1971), and Painter (1979). Until recently, palatography has not been widely used in the study of disordered speech, but recent studies by Hardcastle and colleagues (for example, Hardcastle, Morgan Barry and Clark, 1985) have shown how useful electropalatography can be in the investigation of certain articulatory problems. However, palatography does have certain disadvantages. Firstly, approximants and vowels are difficult to examine, as they involve little or no palate contact. Likewise labial and pharyngeal or glottal sounds cannot be fully examined. Also both direct and indirect palatography are invasive, and thus produce artificiality into the production of utterances by the subject.

Another aspect of articulation investigated by phoneticians is the muscular activity involved in speech production. This has been investigated through electromyography (see descriptions in Keller, 1971; Painter, 1979; and Moore, 1984). This method uses electrodes (either surface or needle) to record the electrical activity of particular muscles and plot the results via a chart recorder (see Tatham, 1984, for a discussion on the accuracy of different chart recorders). From this information a picture can be built up of how particular aspects of speech are controlled by muscular activity. This is of importance for certain types of speech disorder; for example, Moore (1984) describes studies in voice disorders, various types of aphasia and fluency disorders.

Perhaps one of the most useful instrumental techniques for investigating articulation is X-radiography. X-ray examinations may be recorded as still, cine or video pictures, and can give detailed information on articulator placement, and if cine or video is used, on the sequencing and interrelation of the movement of various articulators. It is true, as Keller (1971) points out, that radiographic techniques can only give a two-dimensional picture of speech activity, and indeed this picture tends to be limited to lateral views, as the jawbone mass restricts clear frontal views. Nevertheless, until the fuller development for phonetics of techniques such as ultrasonics, stroboscopy and nuclear magnetic resonance, radiography is perhaps the best means of examining articulation in detail. Ball (1984) describes its application in speech pathology, but a development combining this technique with laryngography is described more fully below. The X-ray microbeam technique (described in detail in Ball, 1984) is presently being further developed for speech pathology in a major project (R. Kent, personal communication), and will eventually have a major role to play in research in our field. Prohibitions of cost, however, effectively rule out microbeam techniques in the area of diagnostics.

A technique on the borderline between articulation and acoustics is aerometry. Simply stated, aerometry investigates air-flow into and out of the oral and nasal cavities, and records measurements via a chart-recorder. Often, a larynx microphone will also be used, and a measurement of vocal cord activity included on the chart. One application of this method, then, could be to measure velopharyngeal opening and closure in both normal and disordered speech (i.e. various type of velopharyngeal inadequacy). An account of its uses in these areas is given in Anthony and Hewlett (1984).

The most important instrumental technique in the description of acoustic events of speech is the sound spectograph (or Sonagraph), which converts an audio input into a hard-copy analysis, in the form of a special paper trace, or 'spectogram'. The analysis most often utilised is of frequency and intensity plotted against time, though the apparatus can investigate other areas such as frequency against intensity. This instrument has been used widely to investigate many aspects of normal and disordered speech, as noted by Painter (1979) and Farmer (1984) respectively. Recent technological advances have increased the usefulness of this approach, as real-time analyses are now possible, as are computerised analyses of spectrograms, greatly increasing accuracy of measurement (R. Kent, personal communication).

Auditory phonetic research has mostly been concentrated on perception. Some of the various instrumental approaches to this area are described in detail in Code and Ball (1984). They have mostly concentrated on the investigation of the perceptual abilities of aphasic patients, and include delayed auditory feedback (Code, 1984a), dichotic listening (Code, 1984b) and time variated speech (Riensche, Orchik and Beasley, 1984).

The remainder of this chapter will review in more detail one instrumental approach that combines two traditional techniques specifically to meet the needs of the speech pathologist.

XERORADIOGRAPHY–ELECTROLARYNGOGRAPHY

I have already briefly referred to the technique of electrolaryngography, itself primarily developed for the investigation of disordered speech (see Fourcin and Abberton, 1971; Fourcin, 1974, 1982; Abberton and Fourcin, 1984). However, here I will examine a development in recent years to investigate voice disorders in particular.

This combined technique is termed 'xeroradiography–electrolaryngography', or XEL for short. The initial descriptions of this approach are found in MacCurtain (1981), Berry, Epstein, Fourcin, Freeman, MacCurtain and Noscoe (1982a), and representative studies are described in Ranford (1982) and MacCurtain and Christopherson (1985). Both Ball (1984) and Abberton and Fourcin (1984) relate XEL to work in radiography and electrolaryngography respectively.

Xeroradiography is an X-radiographic method utilising a special electrically charged plate, which avoids the need for using a photographic chemical plate. Berry *et al.* (1982a) note that xeroradiography was chosen 'for its characteristic clarity of soft tissue detail obtained at low cost in X-ray dose; even individual muscle groups can be detected' (p. 69). The combination of this technique with electrolaryngography 'provides anatomical and functional evidence of soft tissue changes throughout the whole of the vocal tract, and demonstrates how aberrant vocal tract movements create aberrant sounds' (pp. 68-9).

The electrolaryngograph utilises small electrodes positioned externally on either side of the thyroid cartilage. A 2 milliamp AC current is passed across the vocal fold area. Conductance increases as the vocal folds approximate to each other; therefore the apparatus presents a measurement of vocal fold activity, this being displayed on an oscilloscope screen.

One of the advantages claimed for XEL is that in most cases the need for direct laryngography (an invasive technique) is avoided. Furthermore, XEL has been developed to be used easily in the clinical situation. To aid the analysis of the xeroradiographs, a set of 17 voice quality parameters has been drawn up (see Berry *et al.*, 1982a, pp. 69-70), which can easily be located on the xeroradiograph.

Ranford (1982) presented a study of a patient suffering from a voice disorder (weak and tense voice quality) previously undetected. The xeroradiographs, together with photographs of the laryngograph wave patterns, demonstrate the differences observed in the patient before and after therapy.

Berry *et al.* (1982a,b) provide further case histories of various types, and more recently MacCurtain and Christopherson (1985) have used the technique to investigate post-laryngectomy patients.

The development of this combined technique was prompted solely by the needs of speech pathologists for a readily available, non-invasive method for examining laryngeal activity. The xeroradiographic aspect of XEL naturally requires the co-operation of hospital radiography departments, which limits its availability somewhat; however interest in this area seems to be increasing as the usefulness of XEL becomes appreciated.

The brief survey of instrumental phonetic description has not claimed to be comprehensive. New instruments are continually being developed, and I have described here only a few of the more long-standing techniques. In time a literature will have built up on these newcomers, and we will know whether instruments such as Visipitch™ are able to take on the role hitherto played by the laryngograph. Until then, the outline given above includes the most used of the techniques utilised by phoneticians and speech pathologists for the description of disordered speech.

CONCLUSION

This chapter has explored the area of phonetic description; that is, ways of accounting for articulatory, acoustic and auditory aspects of speech events. In particular, it has been concerned with how the needs of speech pathology, and in some cases the information provided by speech pathology, have aided the development of phonetic description.

In many cases speech pathologists will want, or need, to rely solely on their own transcriptional abilities by utilising an impressionistic symbol system. As we have seen, they now have the ability to represent, through symbol systems, not only the full range of normal speech sounds, but a substantial selection of non-normal sounds as well. Further developments in this area are to be expected, with various competing systems being refined, until we can agree on a standard.

In those instances where an impressionistic transcription is not sufficient for purposes of description or of research, speech pathologists now have available a wide range of instrumentation. Many aspects of the production, transmission and reception of speech can be investigated in detail via these instruments, and certain developments in experimental phonetics can be directly attributable to the needs of speech pathology. It is true, of course, that many clinicians do not have ready access to many (if any) of these instruments, and future developments in this field must surely be directed at finding ways of widening this access, as well as developing new and better machinery.

Phonetics and speech pathology are, then, in an on-going mutually supportive relationship. The role of phonetics is no longer a static one: the simple teaching of normal articulation and transcription. In both instrumental and traditional description, phonetics has aided the understanding of speech pathologists of the process of speech production, and the needs and experiences of speech pathologists has prompted exciting developments within phonetic description.

NOTES

1. See further discussion in Code and Ball (Chapter 7, this volume).
2. The group stress that these symbols are *additional* to the IPA. 'They are for use with the IPA alphabet. It should be noted, however, that although they are recommended by the PRDS Group, they are not officially recognised by the IPA' (PRDS, 1980, p. 216).
3. It is true that the voicelessness diacritic, and the dental place of articulation diacritic, are exceptions to this.
4. Surely [L] is an unfortunate choice, as it is often used as a cover symbol for liquids? Superscript [L] is also found for lateral release of plosives.

REFERENCES

Abberton, E. and Fourcin, A. (1984) Electrolaryngography. In Code and Ball (1984)
Anthony, J. and Hewlett, N. (1984) Aerometry. In Code and Ball (1984)
Bailey, C-J.N. (1985) *English phonetic transcription*, University of Texas, and Summer Institute of Linguistics, Arlington

Ball, M.J. (1984) X-ray techniques. In Code and Ball (1984)

Ball, M.J. (in preparation) *Welsh Phonetics*

Ball, M.J., Duckworth, M. and Munro, S.M. (1984) Transcription of disordered phonology in Welsh. *Cardiff Working Papers in Linguistics, 3*, 21-30

Berry, R.J., Epstein, R., Fourcin, A., Freeman, M., MacCurtain, F. and Noscoe, N. (1982a) An objective analysis of voice disorder. Part One. *British Journal of Disorders of Communication, 17*, 67-76

Berry, R.J., Epstein, R., Freeman, M., MacCurtain, F. and Noscoe, N. (1982b) An objective analysis of voice disorder. Part Two. *British Journal of Disorders of Communication, 17*, 77-85

Canepari, L. (1983) *Phonetic notation — La notazione fonetica*, Cafoscarina, Venice

Carney, E. (1979) Inappropriate abstraction in speech-assessment procedures. *British Journal of Disorders of Communication, 14*, 123-35

Code, C. (1984a) Delayed auditory feedback. In Code and Ball (1984)

Code, C. (1984b) Dichotic listening. In Code and Ball (1984)

Code, C. and Ball, M.J. (1984) (eds) *Experimental clinical phonetics*, Croom Helm, London (Published in USA as *Instrumentation in speech-language pathology*, College Hill Press, San Diego)

Farmer, A. (1984) Spectrography. In Code and Ball (1984)

Fourcin, A. (1974) Laryngographic examination of vocal fold vibration. In B. Wyke, (ed.), *Ventilatory and phonatory control systems*, Oxford University Press, London

Fourcin, A. (1982) Laryngographic assessment of phonatory function. In C.K. Ludlow, (ed.), *Proceedings of the Conference on the Assessment of Vocal Pathology*, Maryland: ASHA Reports, *11*

Fourcin, A. and Abberton, E. (1971) First applications of a new laryngograph. *Medical and Biological Review, 21*, 172-82

Grunwell, P. (1982) *Clinical phonology*. Croom Helm, London (2nd edn, 1987, Croom Helm, London/Williams & Wilkins, Baltimore)

Grunwell, P. (1985) Comment on the terms 'phonetics' and 'phonology' as applied in the investigation of speech disorders. *British Journal of Disorders of Communication, 20*, 165-70

Hardcastle, W.J., Morgan Barry, R.A. and Clark, C.J. (1985) Articulatory and voicing characteristics of adult dysarthric and verbal dyspraxic speakers: an instrumental study. *British Journal of Disorders of Communication, 20*, 249-70

Hewlett, N. (1985) Phonological versus phonetic disorders: some suggested modifications to the current use of the distinction. *British Journal of Disorders of Communication, 20*, 155-64

Keller, K.C. (1971) *Instrumental articulatory phonetics: an introduction to techniques and results*, Summer Institute of Linguistics, University of Oklahoma

Koenig, W., Dunn, H.K. and Lacey, L.Y. (1946) The sound spectrograph. *Journal of the Acoustical Society of America, 17*, 19-49

Ladefoged, P., Cochran, A. and Disner, S. (1977) Laterals and trills. *Journal of the International Phonetic Association, 7*, 46-54

MacCurtain, F. (1981) Pharyngeal factors influencing voice quality.

Unpublished PhD thesis, University of London

MacCurtain, F. and Christopherson, A. (1985) Aspects of vocal efficiency in laryngectomy procedures: a pilot study. *CST Bulletin*, *403*, 8-9

Milroy, L. (1985) Phonological analysis and speech disorders: a comment. *British Journal of Disorders of Communication*, *20*, 171-9

Moore, W.H. Jr. (1984) Electromyography. In Code and Ball (1984)

Painter, C. (1979) *An introduction to instrumental phonetics*, University Park Press, Baltimore

PRDS (1980) Progress report. *British Journal of Disorders of Communication*, *15*, 215-20

PRDS (1983) The phonetic representation of disordered speech. *King's Fund Project Paper*, *38*

Principles of the IPA (1949) International Phonetic Association, London

Principles of the IPA, revised edition (1979) International Phonetic Association, London

Ranford, H.J. (1982) 'Larynx-NAD'? *CST Bulletin*, *359*, 5

Riensche, L.L., Orchik, D.J. and Beasley, D.S. (1984) Time-variated speech. In Code and Ball (1984)

Tatham, M.A.A. (1984) Recording and displaying speech. In Code and Ball (1984)

Wood, S. (1982) X-ray and model studies of vowel articulation. *Lund University Department of Linguistics Working Papers*, *23*

9

Theoretical Linguistics and Clinical Assessment

John H. Connolly

INTRODUCTION

During the past 20 years or so there has been a dramatic development in the degree of linguistic sophistication found in the assessment materials available to speech clinicians. Perhaps the most obvious contribution which linguistics has made in this respect lies in the provision of suitable analytical frameworks for the description of clients' language disabilities, and thus it may appear that the benefits which have consequently accrued are due mainly to the clinical application of descriptive rather than theoretical linguistics. Nevertheless, it is unquestionably the case that theoretical linguistics has had, and will continue to have, a part to play in the development of clinical assessment materials, and it is this role that will be the concern of the present chapter.

Theoretical linguistics admits of both direct and indirect applications to clinical assessment. Direct applications exist where particular concepts are taken over as design principles for the construction or interpretation of assessment procedures. As for indirect applications, these occur through the clinical utilisation of descriptive linguistics referred to above, inasmuch as the frameworks and categories of descriptive linguistics rest ultimately upon the foundations of theoretical linguistics. Both kinds of application will be mentioned in the present chapter, but we shall concentrate mainly upon applications of the direct type.

LANGUAGE AND MEDIUM

One of the most fundamental conceptual dichotomies in linguistic science is that between language and the medium in which it is embodied when used in communication; see further Abercrombie (1967, pp. 1-4) and cf. Saussure (1966, pp. 111-22). As far as clinical assessment is concerned, the major consequence of this dichotomy lies in the recognition of a sharp distinction between phonetic and linguistic analysis. In principle this distinction is clear enough, but in practice, as anyone who has taught the subject knows, the theoretically vital difference between phonetic analysis and linguistic analysis at the phonological level is less than self-evident to many people! The traditional tendency in speech pathology to distinguish between speech disorders and language disorders is rather unhelpful in this respect, since it leaves phonological disorders awkwardly straddling the gap and not falling tidily into either category; cf. Crystal (1980, pp. 124-6). However, in recent work on clinical assessment, such as Grunwell (1985), it is recognised that phonological and phonetic disorders represent distinguishable types of disability and that phonological and phonetic assessment accordingly represent separate procedures.

The distinction between phonological and phonetic assessment is an important one from the practical point of view because these two types of assessment focus on quite different aspects of the client's speech. Phonetic assessment is concerned with the client's speech production ability and thus seeks to establish the range of sounds which he is physically capable of uttering. Phonological assessment, on the other hand, addresses the way that he organises these sounds into functional systems of contrast, and combines them into structures, as a basis for communication. Discovering whether a particular client's problems are phonetic or phonological in nature (or both) is essential to the design of appropriate programmes of remediation.

Parallel to the phonological–phonetic distinction in the spoken language is the graphological–graphetic distinction in the written language (cf. Crystal, 1981, p. 197). Speech therapists tend, understandably, to focus their attention more on clients' speech than on the latter's writing ability, with the result that the advances that have been made in clinical phonological and phonetic assessment have not been accompanied by corresponding advances in clinical graphological and graphetic assessment. Perhaps these will come as a future development. If they do, then the language–medium distinction will need to be taken into account there just as carefully as in the devising of assessment procedures relating to the spoken language.[1]

LEVELS OF LINGUISTIC ANALYSIS

Another basic principle of linguistic theory is that language can be analysed at various structural levels or layers. Admittedly, there is not universal agreement as to how many levels need to be recognised, or what they should be called, but no-one denies that a multi-level view of language is well-founded. Indeed, such is the complexity of language that it would be impractical to attempt to describe it without some kind of separation of levels, and this is just as true in clinical linguistics as in any other branch of the subject. Not surprisingly, therefore, a multi-level view of language is generally taken for granted in work in clinical assessment.

At least three distinct levels of linguistic analysis can be identified in relation to the spoken language: the phonological, the grammatical and the semantic. (The term 'grammatical' is used here, as in Crystal's clinical linguistic framework (1980, p. 46), in its narrower sense of 'morphosyntactic'.) Increasingly, however, the description of meaning is being seen as spread between semantics and pragmatics, to the extent that it now seems appropriate to regard pragmatics as a further level of analysis; cf. Levinson (1983, pp. 33-5). If semantics and pragmatics are taken as distinct levels, then pragmatics is seen as relating to those aspects of meaning that are context-specific, for example the reference of pronouns like *I*, *you*, *he* or *she*, whose precise meaning depends on the setting, and which are not properly interpretable out of context.

Assessment procedures are now available in respect of each of the different levels mentioned above, though at present some levels are better catered for than others. Segmental phonology is particularly well served, with many schemes having been put forward, including several fairly comprehensive ones; see especially Ingram's analytical procedures (1981), Crystal's PROPH (1982) and Grunwell's PACS (1985). Non-segmental phonology, on the other hand, is far less well supplied with systematised assessments. The appearance of Crystal's PROP (1982) has ameliorated the situation considerably, but even PROP is somewhat selective in its coverage; cf. Connolly (1983). With regard to the grammatical level, a number of linguistically based assessment procedures have been devised, for example Engler, Hannah and Longhurst's LASS (1973), Muma's CORS (1973), Dever and Baumann's ISCD (1974), Lee's DSA (1974), Crystal, Fletcher and Garman's LARSP (1976), Bickerton's matrix-based scheme (1980) and Miller's ASS procedure (1981). The semantic level, by contrast, is far less well provided for, though the arrival on the scene of Crystal's PRISM-L and PRISM-G (1982) has again improved the position, while Lund and Duchan (1983, pp. 164-222) also contains useful ideas.

As for the pragmatic level, this layer of analysis embraces a rather diverse set of phenomena, even though all of the latter relate in some way to the use of language in context. A thoroughgoing assessment of pragmatic ability might reasonably be expected to embrace the following areas:

(a) The intelligible signalling of the intended meaning to the hearer.
(b) The management of discourse, subdivided into two aspects: (i) textual; (ii) interactive.
(c) The relationship of language to the extralinguistic universe, subdivided into two aspects: (i) reference; (ii) style.
(d) The relationship of language to its paralinguistic and non-linguistic accompaniments.

Let us consider these areas in turn. Intelligibility testing (1a) has a long history, not only in speech therapy but also in other fields, such as language teaching, psychoacoustics, audiology and telecommunications; see, for example, Olsson (1977), Speaks and Trooien (1974), Kyle (1977), Richards (1973, pp. 112-223). Within the field of speech therapy, intelligibility assessment procedures have been devised by, for example, Yorkston and Beukelman (1981) and Weiss (1982), and in addition the research literature contains numerous accounts of intelligibility testing. For further discussion see Connolly (1986).

Discourse (b) has been the subject of considerable theoretical advances in recent years, and the influence of this progress has been felt in the clinical field as well, where clients' ability to manage discourse structure has become a topic of widespread interest. In relation to both theory and clinical application it is convenient to identify two aspects of discourse, as indicated above — namely the textual and the interactive. The textual aspect covers matters such as coherence, cohesion and the organisation of the message; see further Halliday and Hasan (1976), de Beaugrande and Dressler (1981), Brown and Yule (1983). The interactive aspect encompasses such subjects as turn-taking, responding, initiating new topics, conversational repair, the use of politeness formulae and other essentially social expressions like greetings and valedictions, and the accomplishment of various types of speech act. Frameworks now exist for the clinical assessment of many of these facets of interactive discourse; see, for example, Lund and Duchan (1983, pp, 67-78), Prutting and Kirchner (1983), Roth and Spekman (1984), McTear (1985, pp. 53-8). It may be noted also that the top part of the Syntactic Profile Chart in LARSP is devoted to the analysis of discourse interaction. As for the textual aspect of discourse, however, this is not addressed in a comprehensive manner by any existing assessment procedure, though Lund and Duchan (1983, p. 78) provide a starting point, in identifying anaphora, cataphora, ellipsis and contrastive stress as particular cohesive devices that are worth assessing.

The relationship of language to the universe outside of language (1c) involves two rather different considerations. One is the client's ability to refer to entities, processes and so forth in specific contexts, while the other is his control of stylistic variants in accordance with the situation of utterance. With regard to the former, the crucial point is that it is one thing to know the meaning of a word or larger linguistic expression, but another to be able to apply it appropriately in the description of some actual state-of-affairs on some specific occasion. (The distinction that is at stake here is between semantic knowledge on the one hand and pragmatic ability on the other.) Furthermore, as has already been pointed out, there are some words, such as *he*, which have no definite (semantic) sense but whose reference is determined by means of pragmatic principles. No assessment procedure for the systematic assessment of referential ability is currently available. True, PRISM is sensitive to the occurrence of deictic terms like *he*, whose interpretation is contextually determined, but deixis is a broad category which extends to a variety of situation-relative items, such as tense markers, and it cannot really be said that deictic reference is comprehensively assessed either by PRISM or by any other procedure. As regards the control of stylistic variants, although this is referred to in, for example, LARSP, once again there is no detailed assessment procedure relating to this facet of language use.

Finally, let us turn briefly to the relationship of language to its paralinguistic accompaniments, such as voice quality, and its non-linguistic accompaniments, such as gesture. Theoretical frameworks exist for the description of both these types of accompaniment; see, for example, Crystal (1969, pp. 132-40) and Argyll (1978, pp. 37-56) respectively. From the clinical point of view, voice quality in particular has been provided with systematised assessment procedures, such as the Vocal Profile Analysis described in Laver, Wirz, Mackenzie and Hiller (1981). From the perspective of linguistic pragmatics, however, what is needed is a systematic means of assessing the client's ability to relate the paralinguistic and non-linguistic accompaniments of speech appropriately to its linguistic form and content in an appropriate way. Recent work such as that seen in Prutting and Kirchner (1983) and in Skinner, Wirz, Thompson and Davidson's Edinburgh Functional Communication Profile (1984) shows that significant progress is being made in this direction, but there is room for a more detailed assessment procedure of general application.

Pragmatics has, in recent years, aroused such a degree of interest within the clinical field that Prutting and Kirchner (1983, p. 29) are led to speak of a 'paradigm shift', and Duchan (1984) to talk to a 'pragmatics revolution'. Further developments in this domain can therefore be confidently expected.

INTER-LEVEL RELATIONSHIPS

The different levels of analysis are interconnected by means of a relationship known as 'realisation' or 'exponence'; cf. Halliday (1961, pp. 270-2). Phonological structures serve to realise (i.e. give more concrete expression to) units at the grammatical level, which in turn realise semantic-level categories. In this context it is also useful to regard phonetics as a level, and to say that phonological units are realised by phonetic-level exponents.

Because of this interrelationship among levels, the presence of an abnormality at one level may have consequences at other levels; cf. Connor and Stork (1972, p. 44). For example, a client who through an articulatory disability is unable to articulate alveolars and pronounces all such target consonants as labials may be said to have a *primary* phonetic disability, but also a *contingent* phonological disability whereby his speech lacks certain phonemic contrasts. Or again, the absence of sibilant fricatives owing to a primary phonological disorder will lead to a contingent grammatical problem in that many plural noun forms will be indistinguishable from the corresponding singular forms. Careful assessment is, therefore, necessary in order to discover the primary level(s) of disability and to recognise contingent effects for what they are. The assessment procedure proposed by Bickerton (1980) is designed with this issue particularly in mind.

SYSTEM AND STRUCTURE

A further basic dichotomy in linguistics is that between system and structure. Co-occurrent (or syntagmatically related) elements form structures, while sets of mutually substitutable (or paradigmatically related) elements that are capable of occupying the same place in a structure form systems; see further Abercrombie (1967, pp. 70-88) and cf. Saussure (1966, pp. 122-7). In practice it has been at the phonological level that most has been made of this dichotomy, though it is in principle applicable to the higher levels as well, and forms a crucial part of the approach to grammar taken by Halliday and his followers; see, for example, Halliday (1976, pp. 101-35), Berry (1975, 1977). In segmental phonology, systems may be characterised in terms of either phonemes or distinctive features, while structure is commonly described on the basis of phoneme combinations within the syllable. The internal structure of the syllable may be characterised in terms either of the gross categories of consonant and vowel (yielding patterns such as CV, CVC and so on) or of specific phonemes or phoneme classes (for example /s/ or fricative), and the phonotactic constraints, which differentiate permissible from impermissible phoneme

195

sequences, may be described on the same basis.

Any segmental–phonological assessment procedure which is intended to be comprehensive must deal adequately both with the paradigmatic and with the syntagmatic axis. The paradigmatic part of the assessment needs to show which of the phonemic contrasts present in the normal adult language are maintained in the client's speech and which are not. Both consonant and vowel systems should be encompassed, and furthermore, since the range of distinctive segments often varies according to structural place (for example syllable-initial or syllable-final position), this syntagmatic factor also needs to be taken into account. In order to provide a complete picture of the client's phonological system, the procedure should indicate not only the set of contrastive segments in each subsystem, but also how the contrasts are organised in terms of features, and should also facilitate a direct comparison with the normal adult system in both these respects. The syntagmatic part of the assessment needs to deal with phenomena such as the omission of terms from structures (as happens, for instance, in cluster reduction or final consonant deletion), the insertion of segments into structures (epenthesis), the transposition (metathesis) of terms, and harmony phenomena, including contiguous and non-contiguous assimilation (Ingram, 1976, p. 35) as well as coalescence (see, for instance, Cruttenden, 1972, p. 33). In addition it is useful to provide an overall statement of the syllable structures found in the client's speech and a note of any combinations of segments which violate the normal phonotactics. All this represents a large amount of information for an assessment procedure to supply, but recent compilations such as PROPH or PACS provide comprehensive frameworks from which it can be derived.

The notions of system and structure have also been incorporated into the non-segmental–phonological assessment procedure PROP. The latter is organised basically around the structural category of the tone unit and the systems of tone and tonicity which operate within it; see further Halliday (1976, p. 101), Crystal (1969, 1982).

Assessment procedures directed at the grammatical level tend to focus on structure rather than on paradigmatic systems. In LARSP, for instance, structure is dealt with in a comprehensive manner, with proper regard being paid to distinctions of sentence-type (declarative, interrogative, imperative and exclamative) and of rank,[2] with clause-internal, phrase-internal and word-internal (i.e. morphological) structure being sharply separated from each other, with the result that the procedure is sensitive to different levels of achievement on the part of the client in these different facets of grammar. On the other hand, existing procedures do not offer equally detailed assessments of paradigmatic grammatical systems such as tense, mood and aspect; see further Connolly (1984).

At the semantic level the PRISM procedure addresses both the paradigmatic and the syntagmatic axis. PRISM-L represents a genuine attempt to assess the client's vocabulary in terms of semantic systems rather than merely as a collection of items, while PRISM-G is concerned with the semantic relationships among co-occurrent elements.

GENERATIVITY

Some three decades have now elapsed since the appearance of Chomsky (1957), during which time the generative approach to language has, as is well known, exerted an enormous influence upon the development of theoretical linguistics. However, the application of the principles of generative linguistics to the design of clinical assessment procedures has made only a limited amount of headway. Perhaps this is not really surprising, since assessment is an intrinsically analytical activity and the analytical and generative approaches tend to be conceived of as opposite in nature. Nevertheless, both the essential idea of generativity[3] and certain of the technical apparatus evolved within generative linguistics have made at least some impression upon the design of assessment schemes for use in speech therapy.

Given that Chomsky has always stressed the centrality of syntax as the basis for the creative use of language, it might have been expected that assessments directed at the grammatical level would have been the most strongly influenced by generative grammar. In fact, however, the tendency has been for grammatical assessment procedures to borrow ideas and techniques from the generative tradition only in so far as they can serve as useful adjuncts to what are otherwise essentially classificatory frameworks. Thus, for instance, LARSP incorporates the concept of recursion, which is presented as the major characteristic of the Stage V structures in the Syntactic Profile (see Crystal *et al.*, 1976, pp. 75-7),[4] but does not employ generative-style rule formulation. Even when authors of procedures do assume the use of rule-based description, as for example in the case of Bickerton (1980), or refer to constructions in transformational terms, as for instance does Muma (1974, p. 343) in his presentation of the CORS procedure, the intention is not that the assessment should yield a complete generative grammar of the client's language (which would be an impractically ambitious goal in any case) but that it should provide an analytical synopsis of his grammatical disability.

The level of analysis where the influence of generative-style formulation has been strongest to date is that of segmental phonology, where rule-based description has, especially since the appearance of Ingram (1976), come to be accepted as one of the standard formats, often being referred to under the title of 'phonological process analysis'. Admittedly, it is not standard generative phonology that has gained the greatest popularity as a framework for clinical assessment, partly because the Chomsky and Halle (1968) features are poorly suited for this purpose; see, for instance, Walsh (1974). However, assessment procedures deriving ultimately from Stampe's (1979) natural phonology have proved quite successful, especially when used in conjunction with other types of approach, as, for instance, in Ingram (1981) or Grunwell (1985). Nevertheless, there is still room for improvements in the technique of rule-based phonological assessment; in particular, the issue of rule-ordering within such descriptions needs to be given more attention than it has received hitherto.

FUNCTIONALITY

One of the most important characteristics of language from the perspective of speech therapy is its functionality (i.e. its capacity for being used purposively). The main purpose for which language is employed is the communication of meaningful messages from speaker (or writer) to hearer (or reader),[5] and the branch of language study which is concerned with this communicative use of language is known as 'functional linguistics'; see further Dik (1978), Foley and van Valin (1984), Halliday (1985).

The reason why the functionality of language is so significant from the clinical point of view is simply that communication is absolutely vital in human society, so that any individual who is unable to communicate adequately with others is bound to be disadvantaged, and because the main general-purpose means of communication used in human society is language, it is plain that linguistic disability represents a real handicap. Moreover, if the disability is severe, then the handicap is likely to be very serious, which is why the provision of speech therapy services is so necessary.

How does linguistic disability impair an individual's capacity to communicate? The key point is that (normal) language makes available a vast range of what may be termed 'functional distinctions'; see further Connolly (1988). An example of a functional distinction at the phonological level is the paradigmatic contrast between /p/ and /b/, which serves to differentiate pairs of words like *pea* and *bee*. Another is the syntagmatic contrast (cf. Connolly, 1980; Jakobson, 1968, p. 70) between the singleton /p/ and the cluster /pl/, where the presence or absence of /l/ distinguishes pairs of words like *pay* and *play*. At the grammatical level, an example of a paradigmatic distinction is the contrast between past and present tense, while an illustration of a syntagmatic distinction is seen in the presence as against the absence of the adverb *off* in a pair of sentences like *Turn the radio* and *Turn the radio off*.

If a client has either lost or failed to acquire certain functional distinctions, then these distinctions are said to be nullified in his particular system. The nullification of functional distinctions is the basic mechanism whereby linguistic disorders impair communication. Suppose, for instance, that a given client does not phonologically distinguish voiced and voiceless plosives, pronouncing both types as voiced in syllable-initial position and both as voiceless in syllable-final position. This situation may result in any of three different types of communication failure. Firstly, it may result in unintelligibility. For example, the client just mentioned will pronounce *pig* as [bɪk]. Suppose now that he does so without contextual support in the presence of a listener who is unfamiliar with his speech, and that as a result the hearer has no idea what he means. In that case the utterance will be unintelligible. Alternatively, suppose that the hearer infers that the speaker intended to say either *pig* or *big*, but is unsure which. In this case, where the hearer succeeds in narrowing down the range of plausible interpretations to a small, finite number, the utterance will not be unintelligible but ambiguous. Thirdly, suppose that the same speaker utters the word *pad* as [bæt]. It is possible in this instance that the hearer will assume that the speaker really means to say *bat*, in which case the utterance will be neither unintelligible nor ambiguous but *illusive* (Connolly, 1986), i.e. it will receive an unambiguous but unintended interpretation.

It is argued in Connolly (1986) that the three types of communication failure just mentioned — namely unintelligibility, ambiguity and illusiveness — are all special cases of a more general phenomenon, called *indeterminability*. Their capacity to cause indeterminability is one of the chief means whereby linguistic disorders give rise to communicative impairment. Of course, indeterminability is by no means unknown when normal speakers communicate, and ambiguity, in particular, is to some extent built into language structure. Nevertheless, the presence of a linguistic disorder which results in the nullification of functional distinctions constitutes an additional, or *supervenient*, source of indeterminability and hence of communication problems.

Although the capacity to cause indeterminability is perhaps the characteristic of linguistic disorders which has the most detrimental effects upon communication, it is not the only way in which they can bring about communicative impairment. Grammatical or lexical deficits can also impose a handicap in so far as they deny the speaker the possibility of expressing his meaning as fully and/or accurately as a comparable normal speaker would be able to. For example, if a speaker cannot combine more than two elements to form an utterance, or has a poor vocabulary for his age and education, then he will not have the capacity to express as wide a range of meanings as he would if he had a normal level of linguistic ability. He may have to omit elements which should preferably have been included in his utterances, or perhaps use a superordinate term where a hyponym would have been more accurate. If, as the result of a linguistic disability, an utterance is produced which is less specific than a normal speaker would have been expected to produce in the same circumstances, then the utterance is said to be *underspecified*; see further Connolly (1988). Underspecification, like indeterminability, is attributable to the nullification of functional distinctions, whether between shorter and longer utterances describing the same state-of-affairs or between hyponymous and superordinate lexical items.

It seems, then, that functional factors, and in particular the nullification of functional distinctions, are of central importance in accounting for the relationship between linguistic disorders and the communicative impairment to which they give rise, whether through indeterminability or through underspecification. Because the nullified distinctions act in this way as potential sources of supervenient indeterminability or underspecification, one would expect assessment procedures to be sensitive to them, in the following way.

A distinction may be nullified through the absence of one or more of its terms from the system, or through the realisation of more than one of its member terms by the same exponent at a lower level. It may also be nullified in practice if at least one of its member terms is realised by a lower-level exponent which is so different from the normal exponent that even though the actual opposition is preserved, the hearer fails to identify the higher-level term of which the lower-level exponent is supposed to be a realisation, and thus fails to identify it differentially in respect of the other possible terms. These, then, are the circumstances which an assessment procedure directed at finding nullified distinctions should be designed to reveal.

It is certainly true that currently available assessments take functional considerations into account to some extent. PRISM-G provides a form of semantic-functional counterpart to LARSP, while at the phonological level an analysis of homophony is included both in Ingram's procedures and in PACS, and PROPH provides for the identification of individual segments which realise a large number of targets. However, no procedure or range of procedures so far proposed offers a full, systematic analysis of the client's set of nullified distinctions, covering all the different levels of linguistic structure.

The identification of nullified distinctions is not all that may be asked of functionally based assessment, however, since not all nullifications are equal in terms of their adverse effect upon communication. The nullification of a distinction with a relatively high functional load is more serious in this respect than one with a relatively low functional yield. Moreover, when target elements are realised by abnormal exponents, the danger that the targets will fail to be identified increases with the target–realisation distance. A thoroughgoing functional assessment would thus include a measure of the relative functional loads of the various nullified distinctions and of target–realisation distances, so that this information could be used in treatment planning, where it would be relevant to prioritisation decisions. Existing assessment procedures are unable adequately to provide such information, but this situation is likely to change at least at the phonological level in the light of recent research; see Leinonen-Davies (1987), Line (1987). Even at the grammatical and semantic levels, some progress appears possible; see further Connolly (1988).

SYSTEM AND BEHAVIOUR

The dichotomy between what Lyons (1977, p. 26) terms language system and language behaviour (cf. Saussure's (1966, pp. 7-17) *langue* and *parole*) is well established in linguistics. The language system is an abstraction, independent of any actual occasion of language use, whereas language behaviour is an observable event and may take the form of producing or perceiving either speech or writing. Language behaviour is thus dependent upon both realisational medium (spoken or written) and mode (expressive or receptive), whereas in most approaches to theoretical linguistics the language system is regarded as not specific to either of these, except in respect of the distinction between phonology in the spoken language and graphology in the written. The representation of the language system as knowledge in the mind of the (idealised) native speaker is termed linguistic competence by Chomsky (1965, p. 4), who refers to language behaviour under the title of linguistic performance.

The data samples in terms of which clinical assessments are conducted are necessarily based on the client's performance. Nevertheless, as Crystal, Fletcher and Garman (1976, p. 36) rightly maintain, assessment procedures should be concerned ultimately with the system that underlies performance. If no system can be discerned, then it is difficult to arrive at a linguistically well-motivated treatment plan. Workers in the field of clinical linguistics are, however, generally prepared to allow for the possibility of different systems underlying receptive and expressive language behaviour; see, for instance, Ingram (1976, pp. 48-50).

Certain assessment procedures, such as Goodglass and Kaplan's Boston Diagnostic Aphasia Examination (1983), encompass both expressive and receptive mode and spoken and written realisational medium by means of separate subtests. Other procedures are more specific; for instance, PACS is devoted to spoken expression only. Yet others are designed to assess one particular form of language behaviour at a time, but are not specific to a single mode or realisational medium. For example, LARSP can in principle be used to assess either input or output speech or writing, though since it is not divided into subtests, separate applications are necessary for each combination of mode and realisational medium that the user wishes to examine. By selecting an appropriate battery of assessments it is possible to identify both the realisational medium and the mode affected in a given client's language disorder.

The above discussion has been couched in terms of the distinction between system and behaviour rather than competence and performance. This is because as soon as one starts dealing with the notion of competence, numerous problems arise. These include such issues as the form of knowledge representation in the human mind; the relationship between Chomskyan idealised competence and the idiolectal competence which real speakers possess; the question of the narrowness of Chomsky's conception of linguistic competence compared with Hymes' (1972) notion of communicative competence; and the debate over whether language loss affects just performance, as Weigl and Bierwisch (1970) contend, or whether competence, too, is vulnerable, as Whitaker (1970) maintains. Space does not allow for an exploration of these issues here. Suffice to say that the problems concerning the concept of competence do not detract from the validity of the basic distinction between language behaviour and the system that underlies it, and that this dichotomy is of undoubted relevance in the clinical field.

THE DEVELOPMENTAL DIMENSION

The distinction between the synchronic and diachronic approaches in linguistics was established by Saussure (1966, p. 81). The term 'diachronic' is usually employed with reference to the historical evolution of languages, but the same idea of development through time is equally applicable to the linguistic history of individual speakers, though in this context the term 'longitudinal' is normally preferred.

The concept of longitudinal description is relevant in two ways to the discussion of clinical assessment. Firstly, it forms the basis of the monitoring of progress in a client's language in response to therapy. Secondly, it is germane to the characterisation of two diagnostic categories which are often used in relation to the assessment of development disabilities, namely delay and deviance.

The fact that language delay is a developmentally based concept is, of course, immediately clear. Slightly less straightforward, however, is the notion of deviance. The main problem here is that not everyone uses the term 'deviance' in the same way. To begin with, it can be applied either to particular utterances, as, for instance, in the usage of Garman (1980, p. 26), or to overall pathological conditions. In the latter case some authors employ it as a synonym for 'disorder' (for example Menyuk, 1964), while others use it in narrower sense, drawing a distinction between deviance and delay; see, for instance, Byers Brown (1976, p. 45), Ingram (1976, p. 98), Cooper, Moodley and Reynell (1978, p. 14), Crystal (1980, pp. 126-7). Deviance in this last sense refers to a specifically developmental linguistic disorder, which is differentiated from delay in that the latter term implies mere immaturity, whereas deviance describes a condition which is incongruent with the normal developmental pattern. It is, of course, this sense of the term 'deviant' that is inherently developmental in its characterisation.

LINGUISTIC VARIATION

Chomsky (1965, p. 3) attempts to define the central concerns of linguistic description in terms of a homogeneous language community, but this is an (intentional) idealisation, which he sees as a practical necessity. In reality, however, language communities tend to be highly heterogeneous, and different varieties of a given language are found side by side. Linguistic variation is generally described with reference to differences in accent, dialect and style. Accent and dialect variation is related to geographical and socioeconomic factors, while style varies according to the situational context and is influenced by considerations such as the subject-matter of the discourse and the relative status of the participants in the interaction; see further Crystal and Davy (1969), Trudgill (1974).

As is well known, members of language communities such as our own tend to harbour different subjective attitudes towards different varieties of the language(s) which they speak, with the standard variety in general enjoying more prestige than the non-standard varieties, which are often regarded as inferior or incorrect. This prescriptive bias in favour of the standard variety is, of course, resisted in linguistic science, where the descriptive approach prevails. Speech therapists, similarly, have to take an objective view of non-standard varieties and when assessing clients' language they have to take care not to confuse non-standard with genuinely abnormal forms.

Despite the undoubted awareness that exists of the phenomenon of linguistic variation, current assessment procedures do not take as much account of it as they might. As far as accent and dialect variation is concerned, the person administering the assessment is expected to take the initiative in adjusting for non-standard targets, while the phenomenon of inherent variability (see Trudgill, 1974, pp. 45-6) gives rise to difficulties which have not yet been adequately resolved. Stylistic variation, again, is recognised as raising certain problems, especially in relation to the fact that the clinic tends to be perceived as a relatively formal setting compared with many other situations in which the client may find himself, and this may well be reflected in the kind of language elicited when assessing a client who has acquired some command of stylistic differentiation; see further Gallagher (1983). However, as noted earlier, there is no detailed assessment procedure directed at the appraisal of the client's ability to select appropriate styles in a range of different situations.

CONCLUSION

It will have emerged from the discussion in this chapter that many principles of theoretical linguistics have been successfully incorporated into clinical assessment procedures, but that in certain areas one may hope to see further progress in the not-too-distant future. Existing procedures already provide useful information on crucial matters such as (a) the level(s) of analysis affected (phonetic, phonological, grammatical, semantic and/or pragmatic), while permitting primary deficiencies to be distinguished from contingent effects; (b) the paradigmatic and syntagmatic aspects of linguistic organisation at the affected level(s), differentiated as necessary according to mode and realisational medium; and (c) in the case of developmental disorders, the respects in which delay or deviance are exhibited. The structural facets of linguistic disorders are thus quite well catered for by available assessments. On the other hand, the relationship between the structure of language and its use as an instrument of communication in social contexts has received less attention in the design of assessment procedures. Further work directed at the functional/pragmatic aspects of clinical assessment is therefore called for, and can be confidently expected to yield valuable benefits.

NOTES

1. It is true, of course, that certain procedures for the assessment of language disorders, such as Schuell (1973), Porch (1974), Whurr (1974), Spreen and Benton (1977), Kertesz (1982) and Goodglass and Kaplan (1983), involve some analysis of the client's written utterances. However, the focus of such analysis tends to be on the latter's higher-level linguistic abilities rather than on his grapheme system, and in so far as the mechanics of writing or orthographic ability are assessed, the degree of analytical sophistication does not approach that which has now been attained in phonological and phonetic assessment.

2. See Halliday (1961, p. 251).

3. Generativity is the property whereby a grammar specifies explicitly, usually by means of a system of rules, the infinite set of well-formed sentences in the language to which it relates.

4. Structures which have the property of recursion are capable of being used repeatedly in the construction of larger units. Co-ordinate clauses, for example, have this property, since sentences of unlimited length may be built up by placing together a succession of such clauses, one after the other.

5. This is not to say, of course, that language is always used as a vehicle of communication. As a symbolic code, human language can be employed for the purpose of processing information, whether for communicative ends or not; cf. Sperber and Wilson (1986, p. 174). Nevertheless, communication remains the major function which language fulfils in human society.

ACKNOWLEDGEMENT

While preparing this paper I have benefited from discussions with Professor Pamela Grunwell, Miss Jennifer Eastwood and Mrs Rae Smith.

REFERENCES

Abercrombie, D. (1967) *Elements of general phonetics*. Edinburgh University Press, Edinburgh

Argyle, M. (1978) *The psychology of interpersonal behaviour*, 3rd edn, Penguin, Harmondsworth

Berry, M.F. (1975) *Introduction to systemic linguistics. 1: Structures and systems*. Batsford, London

Berry, M.F. (1977) *Introduction to systemic linguistics. 2: Levels and links*. Batsford, London

Bickerton, K. (1980) Working without LARSP. *Working Papers of the London Psycholinguistics Group, 2*, 4-16

Brown, G. and Yule, G. (1983) *Discourse analysis*. Cambridge University Press, Cambridge

Byers Brown, B. (1976) Language vulnerability, speech delay and therapeutic intervention. *British Journal of Disorders of Communication, 11*, 43-56

Chomsky, N. (1957) *Syntactic structures*, Mouton, The Hague

Chomsky, N. (1965) *Aspects of the theory of syntax*, MIT Press, Cambridge, Mass.

Chomsky, N. and Halle, M. (1968) *The sound pattern of English*, Harper & Row, New York

Connolly, J.H. (1980) An explanatory role for linguistics in relation to speech therapy. *Belfast Working Papers in Language and Linguistics, 4*, 85-98

Connolly, J.H. (1983) Review of Crystal (1982). *British Journal of Disorders of Communication, 18*, 130-5

Connolly, J.H. (1984) A commentary on the LARSP procedure. *British Journal of Disorders of Communication, 19*, 63-71

Connolly, J.H. (1986) Intelligibility: a linguistic view. *British Journal of Disorders of Communication, 21*, 371-6

Connolly, J.H. (1988) Functional analysis and the planning of remediation. In Grunwell, P. and James, A. (eds), *The Functional Evaluation of Language Disorders*, Croom Helm, London

Connor, P. and Stork, F.C. (1972) Linguistics and speech therapy: a case study. *British Journal of Disorders of Communication, 7*, 44-8

Cooper, J., Moodley, M. and Reynell, J. (1978) *Helping language development: a developmental programme for children with early language handicaps*, Edward Arnold, London

Cruttenden, A. (1972) Phonological procedures for child language. *British Journal of Disorders of Communication, 7*, 30-7

Crystal, D. (1969) *Prosodic systems and intonation in English*,

Cambridge University Press, Cambridge

Crystal, D. (1980) *Introduction to language pathology*, Edward Arnold, London

Crystal, D. (1981) *Clinical linguistics*, Springer Verlag, Vienna

Crystal, D. (1982) *Profiling linguistic disability*, Edward Arnold, London

Crystal, D. and Davy, D. (1969) *Investigating English style*, Longman, London

Crystal, D., Fletcher, P. and Garman, M. (1976) *The grammatical analysis of language disability*, Edward Arnold, London

De Beaugrande, R. and Dressler, W. (1981) *Introduction to text linguistics*, Longman, London

Dever, R.B. and Bauman, P.M. (1974) Scale of children's clausal development. In T.M. Longhurst (ed.), *Linguistic analysis of children's speech: readings*. MSS Information Corporation, New York

Dik, S.C. (1978) *Functional grammar*, North-Holland, Amsterdam

Duchan, J.F. (1984) Language assessment: the pragmatics revolution. In R.C. Naremore (ed.), *Language sciences: recent advances*, College Hill Press, San Diego

Engler, L.F., Hannah, E.P. and Longhurst, T.M. (1973) Linguistic analysis of speech samples: a practical guide for clinicians. *Journal of Speech and Hearing Disorders*, *38*, 192-204

Foley, W.A. and van Valin, R.D. (1984) *Functional syntax and universal grammar*, Cambridge University Press, Cambridge

Gallagher, T.M. (1983) Pre-assessment: a procedure for accommodating language use variability. In Gallagher and Prutting (1983)

Gallagher, T.M. and Prutting, C.A. (eds) (1983) *Pragmatic assessment and intervention issues in language*, College-Hill Press, San Diego

Garman, M. (1980) Using LARSP in assessment and remediation. In F.M. Jones (ed.) *Language disability in children*. MTP Press, Lancaster

Goodglass, H. and Kaplan, E. (1983) *The assessment of aphasia and related disorders*, 2nd edn, Lea & Febiger, Philadelphia

Grunwell, P. (1985) *PACS: phonological assessment of child speech*. NFER-Nelson, Windsor/College-Hill Press, San Diego

Halliday, M.A.K. (1961) Categories of the theory of grammar. *Word*, *17*, 241-92

Halliday, M.A.K. (1976) English system networks. In G. Kress (ed.), *Halliday: system and function in language*. Oxford University Press, London

Halliday, M.A.K. (1985) *An introduction to functional grammar*, Edward Arnold, London

Halliday, M.A.K. and Hasan, R. (1976) *Cohesion in English*, Longman, London

Hymes, D. (1972) On communicative competence. In J.B. Pride and J. Holmes (eds), *Sociolinguistics*, Penguin, Harmondsworth

Ingram, D. (1976) *Phonological disability in children*, Edward Arnold, London

Ingram, D. (1981) *Procedures for the phonological analysis of children's language*, University Park Press, Baltimore

Jakobson, R, (1968) *Child language, aphasia and phonological universals*, Mouton, The Hague

Kertesz, A. (1982) *The Western Aphasia Battery*, Grune & Stratton, Orlando, Florida

Kyle, J.G. (1977) Audiometric analysis as a predictor of speech intelligibility. *British Journal of Audiology*, *11*, 51-8

Laver, J., Wirz, S., Mackenzie, J. and Hiller, S. (1981) A perceptual protocol for the analysis of vocal profiles. *University of Edinburgh Department of Linguistics Work in Progress*, *14*, 139-55

Lee, L.L. (1974) *Developmental sentence analysis: a grammatical assessment procedure for speech and language clinicians*, Northwestern University Press, Evanston

Leinonen-Davies, E.K. (1987) Assessing the functional adequacy of children's phonological systems. Unpublished PhD thesis, Leicester Polytechnic

Levinson, S. (1983) *Pragmatics*, Cambridge University Press, Cambridge

Line, P. (1987) An investigation of auditory distance. Unpublished MPhil thesis, Leicester Polytechnic

Lund, N.J. and Duchan, J.F. (1983) *Assessing children's language in naturalistic contexts*. Prentice-Hall, Englewood Cliffs, NJ

Lyons, J. (1977) *Semantics*, vol. 1, Cambridge University Press, Cambridge

McTear, M. (1985) *Children's conversation*, Blackwell, Oxford

Menyuk, P. (1964) Comparison of grammar of children with functionally deviant and normal speech. *Journal of Speech and Hearing Research*, 7, 109-21

Miller, J.F. (1981) *Assessing language production in children: experimental procedures*, University Park Press, Baltimore

Muma, J.R. (1973) Language assessment: the co-occurring and restricted structure procedure. *Acta Symbolica*, *4*, 12-29

Olsson, M. (1977) *Intelligibility: an evaluation of some features of English produced by Swedish 14-year-olds*. Acta Universitatis Gothoburgensis, Gothenburg

Porch, B.E. (1974) *Porch index of communicative ability in children*, Consulting Psychologists Press, Palo Alto, California

Prutting, C.A. and Kirchner, D.M. (1983) Applied pragmatics. In Gallagher and Prutting (1983), pp. 29-64

Richards, D.L. (1973) *Telecommunication by speech: transmission performance of telephone networks*, Butterworths, London

Roth, F.P. and Spekman, N.J. (1984) Assessing the pragmatic abilities of children: Part 1. Organisational framework and assessment parameters. *Journal of Speech and Hearing Disorders*, *49*, 2-11

Saussure, F. de, (transl. Baskin, W.) (1966) *Course in general linguistics*. McGraw-Hill, New York

Schuell, H. (1973) *Differential diagnosis of aphasia with the Minnesota test*, revised edn, Oxford University Press, London

Skinner, C., Wirz, S., Thompson, I. and Davidson, J. (1984) *Edinburgh functional communication profile*, Winslow Press, Winslow, Bucks

Speaks, C. and Trooien, T.T. (1974) Interaural alternation and speech intelligibility. *Journal of the Acoustical Society of America, 56,* 640-4

Sperber, D. and Wilson, D. (1986) *Relevance: communication and cognition,* Blackwell, Oxford

Spreen, O. and Benton, A.L. (1977) *Neurosensory center comprehensive examination for aphasia,* revised edn, University of Victoria, Victoria, British Columbia

Stampe, D. (1979) *A dissertation on natural phonology,* Garland, New York

Trudgill, P. (1974) *Sociolinguistics: an introduction,* Penguin, Harmondsworth

Walsh, H. (1974) On certain practical inadequacies of distinctive feature systems. *Journal of Speech and Hearing Disorders, 39,* 32-41

Weigl, E. and Bierwisch, M. (1970) Neuropsychology and linguistics: topics of common research. *Foundations of Language, 6,* 1-18

Weiss, C.E. (1982) *Weiss intelligibility test,* C.C. Publications, Tigard, Oregon

Whitaker, H.A. (1970) Linguistic competence: evidence from aphasia. *Glossa, 4,* 46-53

Whurr, R. (1974) *An aphasia screening test,* University of Reading, Reading, England

Yorkston, K.M. and Beukelman, D.R. (1981) *Assessment of intelligibility of dysarthric speech,* C.C. Publications, Tigard, Oregon

10

Pragmatics and Speech Pathology

Rae Smith

REMEDIAL ISSUES

Over the past 40 years the concern of those involved in treating communicative disorders has ranged over voice, pronunciation, fluency, vocabulary, grammar and alternatives to speech. Throughout this period the central importance of communication and the individual's interactive requirements has remained clear to the majority of clinicians. However, under the influence of linguistic science and the pressure for accountability, speech and language-centred approaches to treatment have sometimes been adopted at the expense of more person-centred ones. When attention is focused on the forms of language rather than upon content and use (Bloom and Lahey, 1978), there is a tendency to disregard textuality in what is taught and to steer the client through a curriculum in a manner which might be expected to induce passivity.

Leonard (1981) found overwhelming evidence in the literature that remedial professionals, hereafter referred to as clinicians, were encountering difficulties in persuading their clients to use in other settings those skills which they appeared to have learned in the classroom or clinic. This failure in skill generalisation provides the impetus for renewed attention to language content and use, and for the incorporation of insights from 'pragmatics' into clinical thinking. Interactive treatment methods clearly need to be developed and evaluated.

At this point it may be helpful to point out that clinicians are likely to exercise considerable caution in altering their professional approach to communicative problems and to highlight some of the reasons for this caution. Firstly, curriculum-centred

treatment is thought to have produced considerable improvement in many clients and, unfortunately, rather little research
evidence is available to support or counter this belief. Secondly,
clinicians are dealing with individuals who are likely to have
encountered failure in interactive situations; therefore it may be
seen as useful to equip them with skills before further interactions fail. Thirdly, communicative failure occurs for a wide
variety of reasons, some of them involving physical structures or
neurological mechanisms and most of them affecting the forms
of speech or language. In these circumstances a mechanistic
approach to treatment could be seen as entirely appropriate. It
will be some time before clinicians can confidently predict
which clients and which types of disorder will most readily
respond to any particular treatment, and in the absence of
conclusive research it would be unwise to abandon approaches
which have met with success, albeit limited (Smith, 1987b).
What is needed is a willingness to test the hypothesis of Snow,
Midkiff-Borunda, Small and Proctor (1984) that more natural,
interactive teaching which actively involves the client may
produce better results. Speech and language clinicians in general
do hold communicative values, and are likely to respond to such
a challenge.

If interactive therapy is to be attempted models will need to
be provided (Hart, 1986); the training of clinicians will have to
include the information that children and others communicate
less readily when authority figures are highly directive (Snow,
1984) and clinicians, psychologists and linguists will need
detailed awareness of the relevance of pragmatics to communicative disorder. With the latter recommendation in mind some
areas of pragmatics are now discussed.

AREAS OF CONSIDERATION

Function

This is a term which poses problems because of the variety of
ways in which it can be used in speech pathology. One reads of
'functional assessment', 'functional disorders', 'disorders of
function', 'functional treatment approaches', etc. In order to
clarify this term it may be helpful to consider several quite
distinct usages:

(1) The social function which an individual is performing in association with the role adopted at any particular time, e.g. 'teaching'; 'helping'; 'debating'.

(2) The function for which language is being employed by the individual or the function of the language itself as described by Dore (1974); Bates, Camaioni and Volterra (1975); Halliday (1975); Tough (1977) — for instance requesting, greeting, protesting, informing. See also 'speech acts', this chapter.

(3) The function of particular grammatical arrangements in the service of meaning as described by Dik (1978) and by Halliday (1985).

(4) The individual's ability to function as assessed by herself and others. In the case of communication this refers to the ability to *use* what she knows in a variety of situations, i.e. 'performance'.

(5) 'Functional disorder', which means in one sense an absence of function but in another sense means an inability to perform certain functions for reasons which are not apparently organic.

(6) Pragmatic functions which we need to perform if satisfactory communication is to take place, e.g. attending, intending, non-verbal supporting, deixis, listening and interpreting, turn-taking, initiating, maintaining or switching topic, monitoring, presupposing, code switching, repairing, use of cohesive devices, closing topic/interaction, temporal integration over long periods. Of these, monitoring has received the least attention. It must be stressed that all parties to an interaction can vary as to the efficiency with which these functions are performed. If attention is focused solely upon the client's need to improve, then the possibility that others, for instance medical staff, are rendering interaction difficult may be missed.

Context

Context is what gives significance to all our experience; for instance an accident which takes place during a rugby match is normally regarded quite differently from an identical incident elsewhere, and a man who says 'This car performs reasonably well', is understood differently when we know whether he is buying or selling.

Using language, or any alternative to speech, in a communicative way involves weighing up the situation, the recipients of the communication, certain areas of shared knowledge and the communicative medium itself, then making choices and putting them into effect. This is a task of considerable complexity which is executed with varying degrees of proficiency by people of differing ability and experience. If these facts are not taken into consideration when assessing and planning treatment for those with communicative disorders, a superficial, de-contextualised view of language and of the person results. Given such a view, assessment will be less realistic and treatment less interesting and, above all, less memorable for the client. Generalisation of what is taught will therefore be less likely. Some types of context which are important for speech pathologists are: the context within which clients are likely to use what is taught; the clinical context, including the personal relationship, within which the teaching takes place; the context in which the language being learnt exists, e.g. a real-life event, a story, a conversation, a game, a song, a joke, an exercise, a list. Little comment is needed as to the memorable and salient qualities of the last two, and yet they are quite frequently employed as teaching contexts (Davis and Wilcox, 1981; Colmar and Wheldal, 1985; Letts, 1985; Panagos, Bobkoff and Scott, 1986).

Consideration should be given to the discourse context of sentences; syntactic context of words; continuous speech context of phonemes (sandhi) and to the communicative context of gestures and intonation patterns, etc., since these alter not only the actions, sounds, words and sentences themselves but in some cases their significance to the learner. Research is needed in this area.

Finally, the influence of context upon assessment should be kept in mind. Individuals who are being assessed are sometimes more aware of the context than is the assessor. Just as the ability to use ellipsis correctly should be regarded as a plus feature, so should the ability to allow for visual context: 'What is he doing?' 'That' is a successful exchange if both people can *see* what he is doing. Also, as clinicians are well aware, clients perform differently in different settings, and it is wise to collect assessment information within a variety of contexts (Sarno, 1969; Holland, 1980; Gallagher, 1983; Tizard and Hughes, 1984).

214

Paralinguistic features

At the beginning of life human infants succeed in communicating with caregivers by means of a variety of cries. Adults and siblings become expert at interpreting the needs and emotions of those in their charge, although intention is sometimes thought not to enter into the baby's activities at this early stage (Piaget and Inhelder, 1969). It is not only the quality of the cry that differs with the child's mood and situation but also such features as attack, length of phonation, body movement and facial expression.

As intentionality develops (Bates, 1974, 1976; Bates *et al.*, 1975; Dore, 1979) infants appear to make use of such abilities as eye pointing, body positioning, arm raising, manipulation of the listener, vague gesturing and facial changing, as well as the progressive differentiation of vocal sound. All these features provide major clues to the child's affect and communicative intention, provided that the partners are alert and imaginative and that they share certain life experiences and cultural observations with the young child.

When intelligible speech is slow to develop considerable communicative success can still be experienced provided that the value of these non-verbal events is acknowledged by all concerned (Leudar, 1981).

Once speech begins these non-verbal activities and events continue to play an important part in the sharing of meanings, though not always by intention, and most of us are alert to this fact, seldom missing the lift of an eyebrow or the mistake in intonation which tells us that a news reader has failed to anticipate correctly the end of a sentence. Teachers and therapists, however, sometimes neglect these important features or assume that such things as intonation and stress can be added as refinements after phonology and syntax have been acquired or re-learnt. Clinical experience suggests, however, that if an interactive approach to therapy is adopted, prosodic features are easily and confidently corrected by patients of all ages, and with a variety of diagnoses, before phonology and syntax are perfected. This appears to assist intelligibility and acceptability. Conversely there have been occasions when people referred part-way through treatment by other methods have proved unable to shake off the stilted and monotonous delivery which accompanied strained attempts at correct production.

Prosodic features and natural gesture form such an important area of pragmatics that it is surprising how infrequently clinical records and research reports make reference to them. Not only would research into the most effective teaching methods for prosody and all gesture, including sign languages, be valuable, but further insight is needed into the deficit of those children, and adults, possibly right hemisphere-damaged, who experience difficulty in spontaneously interpreting or making use of them. For linguists this might involve examining further the systematicity of para-language and seeking answers to such questions as what is it that enables young children to understand others with supposedly 'unintelligible' phonology or, conversely,why is it that some phonologically adequate speech is still unintelligible? Maasen (1986), and Connolly (1986), have usefully discussed intelligibility.

The given and the new

Talking to an old friend, as we all know, is quite different from talking, even on the same topic, with a stranger. Shared knowledge from earlier stages of the friendship enables us to understand the significance attached to certain words and phrases and to guess at implied meanings on the basis of the sketchiest of utterances, e.g.:

'It went again.'
'Why this time?'
'The usual.'

Not only is exact reference unnecessary, but the friendship is confirmed by its omission.

Shared culture, subculture, experience, education and language enable us to make assumptions not only about what people mean by what they say, but about what a listener will understand from the language we use ourselves. We assume, for instance, that 'monotony' and 'sadistics' refer to Monopoly and statistics without an explanation on the part of even the first person who uses the joke form, but sometimes fail to explain familiar words such as 'wellies' to visitors from California who are thus mystified. It is all too easy to credit others with information they do not possess or, conversely, to burden them with

216

superfluous explanations, 'Thank you mother, I *know* that'.

This balancing of presuppositions is one of the major skills involved in successful communication. From complex decisions such as whether or not to remind Charlie that Helen is Kathy's daughter; the one who went to France and he met the Christmas before last, or simply to use the name Helen; to the apparently simple one of whether it would be appropriate to use 'a house' or 'the house', the skill is that of putting one's self in the position of the other person and then mobilising the linguistic knowledge that enables one to signal 'I know that you know that we both know X.'

To regard this complex issue as one involving only surface forms of language, and to teach it as such, would be to neglect the helpful interactional cues which alert people to what can be regarded as 'given' and what must be treated as 'new'. On the other hand some clients do appear to lack knowledge of which surface forms their listeners are likely to expect in particular circumstances; therefore it should be helpful to explore whether, and when, the use of prompting, modelling or explanation as to precisely which details are required by the listener is desirable; also whether some more indirect means of clarifying what is needed, and why, could be devised. The advantage of the latter would be that rather than placing a requirement upon clients it would enable them to provide improvements of their own volition. Even phonological corrections can be achieved in this way.

Clients who have difficulty with the given and the new are people suffering from aphasia or autism; some dysfluent people and the developmentally delayed (De Hart and Maratsos, 1984).

It has been suggested (Baron-Cohen, Leslie and Frith, 1985) that autistic people in particular experience this difficulty, because they lack a 'theory of mind' which would enable them to tell themselves what the communicative partner is thinking; this suggests that one might consider describing one's thoughts and communicative needs to them. Problems of attention and comprehension would be anticipated by many clinicians; however, this does appear to be an approach that should be attempted and researched with all groups who experience difficulty with imagining the thoughts and feelings of others, including socially incompetent adults.

Deixis

Deixis means pointing; virtually saying to one's self 'Here am I; here I stand; this is now; other people and objects are not me; other places are not here; other times are not now.' Young children quickly learn to think deictically and to indicate linguistically which elements of the not here, not now and not me they are considering.

For some children, however, tasks of a deictic nature remain problematic, particularly those involving reference to persons. These children, especially the autistic, appear to find it difficult to have a clear view of themselves, are disorientated or cannot grasp the linguistic means of indication. Adults suffering from disorientation, dementia and aphasia may also experience some degree of deictic confusion, or may not have access to the requisite linguistic forms. In order to appreciate the importance of deixis imagine discussing how to collect someone from a train without using the words he, she, him, her or any that refer to time or place. 'This', 'that', 'these', 'those', are not particularly important when people are together in the same activity and can physically point to what they are interested in, but small words of this kind gain in importance when non-verbal communication does not form part of the interaction and are culturally expected even when it does. Deictic terms make story-telling possible, enable us to make arrangments, facilitate the giving and receiving of instructions, directions and advice and enable us to establish a joint focus of attention with communicative partners. Thus anyone lacking the ability to think deictically or to comprehend or convey deixis linguistically is likely to appear unco-operative or fundamentally uncommunicative. Without the ability to indicate, how is it possible to share one's opinions or wishes? Small children can be observed physically pointing by a variety of means at an early stage in development and an alert care-giver, sibling or clinician can do much to foster interactive skills by responding to these non-verbal signals or to a repetitive 'dat' 'dat'. Appropriate responses include naming, playing with or passing the object, engaging in object-permanence games such as hide-and-seek or peekaboo, exclaiming at the beauty, surprisingness, dirtiness, etc. of the focus of attention 'Oh that's a lovely doggie', 'Oh he's all muddy', 'Where's it gone? Down there', etc. Developmentally young people will often indicate interests in this way either non-verbally, by means of proto-words or by minimal utterances such as 'Wan uh'. Research by now suggests (Wells, 1981; Snow *et al.*, 1984) that teachers, care-givers and clinicians would be wise at least to test the hypothesis that it is more facilitative of communicative development to respond to these early deictic acts by means of contingent remarks or co-operative actions than to attempt to teach deixis by means of 'Show me ...' therapy. The crucial difference is that the person with most to learn is in charge of the choice of focus and may consequently be motivated, alert and retentive. This does not mean that the child or mentally handicapped client has taken charge in every respect; only that a process of negotiation has begun. Negotiation is crucial for the development of interactive ability, as is intersubjectivity, therefore clinicians wearying of pushing someone round and round a room in response to 'Want it horsie. Want it horsie 'gen' have every right to contribute 'No more. I'm tired' or 'Well just one more then.' This does not take the initiative away from the client, but neither does it teach her to ignore the communicative partner's humanness (Smith, 1987a).

Referents coexisting in the minds of the individuals in communication and in the physical world are an important feature of deixis. Fillmore (1975) pointed out that no-one would be able to understand a message floating in a bottle in mid-ocean which read 'Meet me here at noon tomorrow with a stick about this long.' The message may be clearly written, the words are familiar, the syntax is adequate but essential knowledge or the means of conveying it is missing; sometimes it is the intersubjectivity which appears to be lacking.

Speech acts

Speech act theory contends, as most ordinary human beings do, that when an utterance is made, something lies behind the words. As children we learn to recognise such activities as 'showing off', 'trying to make you feel better', 'sucking up to teacher', 'putting you on', 'winding you up', etc. Our family and peers put us wise to these things little by little until we are in a position to define activities for ourselves. Individuals may not agree in their interpretation; for instance the wolf's friendly greeting would be viewed rather differently by Red Ridinghood; readers of the story and, had she only been present, Red

Ridinghood's mother. Our interpretations depend upon experience, information and viewpoint. Mother has experience, though hers may differ from that of her growing offspring, giving rise to disagreement. Daughter and reader of the story have information, though to varying degrees; she has been warned but has not understood the full import of the information; we may have heard something about wolves already, peeped at the book's later pages or read the story before.

An utterance, then, has meaning beyond the dictionary definition of the words used, and even beyond our interpretation of their syntactic arrangement; for instance, not only will jazz buffs understand, at the discourse level, that expressions such as 'She plays a mean trumpet' signify approval, but they will also be able to interpret the use of such expressions within a social context to perform speech acts, e.g. flattering, identifying, joking or claiming status. Human intercourse depends, to a greater extent than is generally acknowledged, upon the ability to perceive speech acts; to reconcile differences in perception and to work with the possibilities created by the interplay of intention and interpretation (Wardhaugh, 1985).

Speech act theorists Austin (1962); Strawson (1964); Grice (1975); Bruner (1975); and Searle (1969, 1975); have explored these issues and Dore (1974); Bates *et al*. (1975); Bates (1976) and Dore (1979); and others have examined the emergence of speech acts in childhood.

From the clinical point of view, speech act theory constitutes a major challenge to the notion that successful communication is simply a matter of uttering, intelligibly, certain grammatically correct language structures. The complexity of the tasks involved in performing and responding to even those basic skills is now well understood but when the content, the manner, the intention, the direct or indirectness and the effect of communications are also taken into consideration, their complexity is seen to be even more prodigious. One way of handling this challenge would be to ignore it. However, the majority of clinicians embraced remedial speech teaching in the first place because of a personal interest in human interaction, and it is well known within the professions concerned that attending only to the forms of speech and language is in the end somewhat demotivating; also it falls short of what many clients appear to need. Not only do those children and adults who are experiencing 'semantic/pragmatic' difficulties (Ochs and Schieffelin, 1979;

Lucas, 1980), require wide-ranging therapy, but the speed of learning and the skill-generalisation of other clients may be improved by working at the discourse level and taking sociolinguistic considerations into account.

Research into these issues is urgently needed if therapy is to become more effective, and the potential contribution of linguistic science to real communication is to be maximised; therefore it may be useful to consider some of the points at which speech act theory and clinical activity intersect.

Social skills are now seen as lacking in many clients with a disability of mind, whether they are categorized as 'autistic', 'disturbed', 'educationally handicapped', 'brain-damaged', 'developmentally delayed' or 'language disordered'. For these client groups interactional skills are currently taught and fostered by many of the professionals concerned with their welfare, though all too often superficial behaviours are imposed upon them in the name of 'social skills training'. Other speech/ language clients may be regarded as socially unskilled; for example some dysfluent people and some of those who experience voice-related problems. Clinicians who assist these people with social interaction may find it helpful to consider whether they are capable of performing a variety of speech acts in a variety of circumstances. If not: which types of speech act would they most like to have at their disposal? Which do they most appear to need? e.g. requesting, questioning, challenging, greeting, persuading. How successfully do they interpret the speech acts of others? Are their attempts at speech act performance appropriate to the situation? Do others misinterpret their attempts? Are there conflicting views as to what is appropriate? Clinicians may also find it useful to consider, as speech act theorists have done, several distinct but coexisting components of the communicative act, for instance the intention behind it; the behaviour by which it is executed, e.g. uttering sounds or words, kicking, signing; the effect it might be expected to have and the effect it actually does have. There is still some way to go before speech act theory becomes totally clear on all these points. McTear (1985a) has suggested that clinical scientists would do well to exercise caution in adopting a theory that is unclear, and Austin (1962) has pointed out that some of the above components of communicative acts are unmistakably linguistic ones, while others, for instance the effect and perhaps the intention of the act, are not necessarily linguistic at all.

221

Despite these difficulties clinicians are likely to remain interested in speech acts since they represent the *raison d'être* of all
speech and language activity.

The interpretation of speech acts may be a problem area for
clients particularly those who have had difficulty in learning to
decode language itself or who do not confidently evaluate
situations or the behaviour of others. We all take time to learn
these evaluative skills; indeed this is one of the problems in
protecting children from abuse or consumers from tricksters,
but there are individuals who fail almost completely to recognise
what is intended or implied by what others say. It is not only
clients, however, who are able to benefit from the examination
of interpretation: relatives, teachers and nursing staff sometimes
construe attempts at improved communication on the part of
people with disabilities as impertinence or rebellion. It can be
extremely helpful to the client in this situation if a clinician is
able to explain that there are other ways of regarding these
attempts to gain independence or improved status. Therapists
too are sometimes apt to interpret initiations or experiments on
the part of their clients as challenges to their authority. An
example of an alternative interpretation follows. A four-year-
old boy, who was reported to be 'difficult and unco-operative'
was asked to think about his unusual phonology. He responded
with 'I talk how I like; no one tells me how to talk.' His therapist
chose to interpret this as 'testing' and therefore responded with
'That's OK really, except just that people can't understand you.'
This prompted a co-operative exchange and, as clinical records
show, rapid resolution of what had appeared to be a serious
speech problem. Similarly a teacher of the deaf reports that a
notoriously unco-operative pupil refused to do the work set and
responded when asked why with 'Because you're too old and
stupid.' This she chose to interpret as 'being deliberately outra-
geous for the purpose of getting a reaction', i.e. as an invitation
to interact; she therefore responded with 'Yes and you are too
young and cheeky.' This resulted in prolonged laughter on the
part of both people and a greatly improved teaching/learning
relationship. Little imagination is required to estimate the
duration of these two problems had the people in question
chosen to escalate the power-based interaction that was being
set up. This brings us to a point raised by Levinson (1983, p.
291),

attempts to bridge the gap (between what utterances 'literally' mean and 'actually' do in the way of actions) with theories of indirect speech acts have provided at best only partial solutions. For questions of context, both sequential (or discourse) context and extralinguistic context, can play a crucial role in the assignment of utterance function.

Levinson goes on to stress the complexity of the inferential process involved, and to remark that the present stage of linguistic theory does not even begin to handle this complexity.

How are we to inform one another of the rules for interpreting and issuing speech acts? We may explain that on this occasion 'Climb up on that wall and jump off Jonesy' constitutes a practical joke, and that the correct playground response to it is something similar to 'Get lost', but does that help the client on the next occasion? As yet we are as far from understanding this as we are from certainty as to the best method of improving syntactic production. However, there is one theorist (Grice, 1975) who has examined what he calls the 'co-operative principle' which operates, or should operate, in social exchanges. He suggests that awareness of certain rules for the success of speech acts enables us not only to perform them but to interpret them. Mistakes are, however, sometimes made because we assume that these rules have been adhered to when they have not. Co-operative behaviour, according to Grice, involves offering the right amount of information for the purpose in hand, attempting to make one's contribution truthful, relevant and adequate. In addition one ought to aim for clarity and as much brevity as is consistent with the above conditions. Clearly these are ideal conditions, which a good many of our interactions do not even approach. Clearly too it will be necessary, on some occasions, to sacrifice one condition to another, and to rely heavily upon contextual factors for the successful completion of a communicative act. Together these conditions are sometimes referred to as 'sincerity' rules, on the basis that a sincere attempt to communicate is being demonstrated. However, this is not particularly helpful as the following examples demonstrate.

'Will I fail or will I pass?'
'Are the pampas birds or grass?'

This is not sincere but it succeeds in communicating anxiety about an examination.

'Get out.'

This is sincere but may fail to achieve its objective since it sets up resistance in the recipient. The rule concerning *relevance*, however, is currently regarded as central to successful performance of speech acts.

In teaching stituations the question of co-operation becomes crucial. The intention of the teacher or clinician is that something shall be attended to, remembered and used at the appropriate time. For this to happen the learner must participate in some way, preferably making the information his/her own and integrating it with other information. If s/he merely agrees to go through the motions of paying attention, something may still be remembered and used, though less vigorously, but if co-operation is completely absent, nothing will be learnt. Teachers and clinicians vary as to the extent of their belief in self-motivated learning and their commitment to interactive methods of teaching (Smith, 1986), but most are aware that in the case of some pupils and clients less than adequate co-operative conditions exist. If only for the purpose of understanding these 'difficult' cases, speech act theory provides a starting point for exploration.

When considering interactions it is important to consider how participants affect one another. Clinicians and researchers may wish to use the framework of speech act theory to describe interactions, but will need to keep in mind Levinson's reservations about the need for extralinguistic information and his plea, responded to by McTear (1985a), for sequential analysis, rather than classification of isolated speech acts. This would mean that rather than observing the type and number of speech acts employed by patients and assigning these to the categories 'appropriate' or 'inappropriate', it would be necessary to observe as far as possible the sequence of events and utterances within which those speech acts occurred. Prutting (1982) also cautions against focusing all our attention on one member of the interactive dyad, but in general this advice has been ignored. Sequential analysis would not only enable us to consider the client's ability to perform and decode speech acts, but would motivate some overdue examination of the language, expectations, attitudes and behaviour of clinicians and teachers. Some of the few studies of clinical interaction so far available are those of Letts (1985), Panagos *et al.* (1986), Ripich, Hambrecht and Panagos (1984) and Ripich and Panagos (1985).

Looked at in this way, speech act theory has a contribution to make to the treatment of dysfluency, voice problems, aphasia, autism, developmental delay and specific developmental language disorders, and those dysarthrias and dyspraxias which call for compensatory strategies. It may also contribute to research, rehabilitation of offenders, social work, counselling and psychotherapy, policing, management, staff relationships and the reduction of marital disharmony and child abuse.

Temporal integration/discourse

Whereas 'pragmatics' is a term used to cover the whole area of language use and communication in action, 'semantics' and 'discourse' studies examine levels of language. The semantic level is that at which the meaning–structure of a language exists; at this level words are defined by the other words we use to describe their meaning and even such things as idioms are fixed in ways which can, again, be verbally described. At the discourse level, however, meanings are far more fluid; at this level we are able to attach to words and to non-verbal communication whatever meaning seems most appropriate to the circumstances in which they are encountered. To do this we mobilise all that we already know about the world, the situation and our communicative partners; we have some choice as to interpretation, and we may choose freely how to encode messages. For instance, if we know our partners well we can expect that some freshly minted expression such as 'Out of the broom cupboard' (Roulstone, 1981) (speech therapists working on real-life communication) will be readily understood. Similarly, by now, many adults know how to interpret broadcasts concerning South Africa which speak of 'Certain events' or 'Certain people whose identity I am not allowed to reveal and whose uniforms I am not at liberty to describe.'

At this level of language, meanings have been negotiated over time and a grammar beyond that of sentences can be shown to exist (Longacre, 1979). In order to function at this level one must be able to retain impressions of what is past and

225

to create, in one's mind, an image of some kind relating to the future. This is the reason why psycholinguists and speech pathologists attach importance to 'object permanence' and related concepts in the study of speech readiness (Ratner and Bruner, 1978; Rice, 1984).

Very young children are able to function at the discourse level, e.g. 'Want it 'gen', but in order to do so they, or their disabled fellows, must at least be able to form the intention to communicate, (Piaget and Inhelder, 1969). An empathic observer, however, can sometimes guess at the thoughts which are not being expressed and model suitable utterances for the uncommunicative partner. This is how conversation begins for many speech-handicapped people, e.g. 'We say "more please"'.

Clients labelled as having 'semantic/pragmatic' disorders (Lucas, 1980; McTear, 1985a,b,c; Haynes, 1986; Conti-Ramsden and Gunn, 1986), are those who have failed to negotiate meanings or to conduct exchanges successfully with those around them, for reasons supposedly other than articulatory, phonological or syntactic ones. Their difficulties often exist, or perhaps become evident, at the discourse level. They are not able to converse satisfactorily, either because they lack the pragmatic or linguistic means or because their own interior discourse is inadequate; for example they make remarks which are not contingent upon what has just been said, and they fail to use cohesive devices or to keep track of what such words as 'it' are likely to mean. The use of silence and pausing behaviour is often problematic in these failed interactions.

Ulatawska, North and Macaluso-Haynes (1981), found that adults suffering from aphasia, unlike psychotic individuals, exhibited relatively intact discourse abilities which could be exploited in the treatment of their syntactic and other difficulties. While pragmatically based treatment approaches have much to recommend them (Wilcox and Davis, 1982), the discourse and pragmatic abilities of aphasic people, especially those suffering right hemisphere damage, would bear further investigation. There is considerable variation within this client group; sometimes communication is less effective than the results of language tests would lead one to expect; sometimes confusion is evident and clients sometimes report loss of interest in such things as newspapers, broadcasts, conversation and correspondence, despite partial recovery from depression and satisfactory performance in tests of sentence construction and comprehension. These issues are of considerable importance when formulating treatment objectives.

Discourse analysis is still at an early stage of development (see Coulthard, 1985), there are considerable problems involved in using even such well-known procedures as that of Sinclair and Coulthard (1975) (cf. Edmondson, 1981); however, clinicians would do well to undertake some analysis of the various interactions attempted by children or adults suspected of pragmatic deficits. This is not suggested as a means of apportioning blame for interactive failures, but as an aid to achieving the high quality of interaction called for in these special circumstances (Panagos *et al.*, 1986).

Two areas of possible research suggest themselves: firstly, discourse comprehension and secondly, discourse and social integration.

Both child and adult clients vary considerably in their ability to interpret new, obscure or indirect communications, and it is not always clear how those who have difficulties at the discourse level can best be helped, or to what extent semantic problems complicate the picture of their disability. It is not even certain that Grice (1975) was correct in thinking that our attempts to understand what is said begin from the supposition that his co-operative maxims have been adhered to by the speaker. So great is the disruption of thinking and deprivation of enjoyment in those who experience comprehension problems that information in this area is urgently required. Research of this nature would also have application to artificial intelligence.

Temporal integration — i.e. continuity of relationships, knowledge of consequences, care for the future and the connection of thought and feeling — plays a part in our ability to function socially. Deficits in this area are thought to contribute to delinquency and behaviour problems (Stott, 1966). Emotions may be, to some extent, mediated verbally, and personal relationships certainly are; therefore it would be well worth investigating the extent to which discourse disability contributes to social malfunction.

Metacommunication

In recent years there has been a growing awareness of the way in which language use affects humankind. The terms 'lack of

227

communication' and 'communication breakdown' have become part of the English-speaking layman's inner language. Consciousness about the sexism of language has been raised to the point where one thinks twice about using 'layman' and certainly would not use 'mankind'. Nobody uses the word 'nigger' any more, other than in very special circumstances: 'white nigger', etc., though many still use the term 'denigrate' without realising how insulting these equations of black with bad can seem to black people. Those who are aware that attitudes of their own have been shaped by language willingly avoid using 'geriatric' to mean disintegrating, or 'spastic' to mean incompetent, but it is usual to deny that the more subtle forms of pejorative language use have any effect at all. Sometimes this attitude can be changed by exercises such as 'For "ladies" read both "ladies" and "gentlemen".'

Awareness of the powerful effect exerted by the choice of words, i.e. metalinguistic awareness, has long been cultivated by special groups such as writers, lawyers, orators and confidence tricksters. The awareness extends to cover all levels of language and is present to some degree in most of us. Individuals commonly help one another with language awarenesss, e.g.:

> 'It isn't "beige"; it's more "cream" or "stone".'
> 'Ask for "*horse* mushrooms".'
> 'Duck when I say "boom coming over".'

Jokes and catch phrases depend sometimes on shared language awareness; e.g.:

> 'Not a lot.'
> 'Mornington croissant.'
> 'What d'you call a man with a spade in his head.'
> 'Doug.'
> 'What d'you call a man without a spade in his head?'
> 'Douglas.'

Some even on knowledge of intonation patterns:

> 'What d'you call a man whose just got out prison?'
> 'Hum'phrey.'

Children enjoy a form of play which involves pushing newly acquired mastery of language forms to the limit:

'Where are you going?'
'Out bom bout tiddle out no fout.'
'Derragid yerragoo terragake marragy beragook.'
'Naygo aygi daygidaynt.'
'Life is butter melon cauliflower.'

or more simply:

'A lemon oh pea.' (l m n o p)

Some children's writers, notably Dr Seuss, exploit this form of
play; as do some, too few, speech clinicians. However, clinicians
do expect a great deal of metalinguistic awareness from their
clients and from their clients' families. Normally this awareness
is very carefully cultivated by means of painstaking exercises,
explanation and demonstration coupled with games of a slightly
different kind from the above, and requests for serious home
practice. Increasingly, motivation is provided by allowing the
original teaching to arise out of a communicative situation in
which the client is genuinely involved; e.g.:

C. '... and beans and sausages and ships and ...'
T. 'Did you know you said ships instead of chips? I'll show
you how to get it right. Let's draw a plate full of ships to
remind us how funny it is.'

or

T. 'Are there any names of your friends that are not very
easy to say? It there one you'd specially like to get right?'

or

T. 'Tell the shop lady "ball please".'

This is known as 'pragmatically orientated' treatment but
involves teaching metalinguistic awareness. 'Metalanguage';
language used to talk about language, is also taught and utilised
by speech clinicians.

Occasionally clinicians fail to appreciate that metalanguage is
beyond their clients' processing ability; this can be true of the
very young, or older brain-damaged or mentally handicapped

people. Metalanguage and metalinguistic awareness can also be unsuspected problem areas for the relatives on whom the client depends for continuity of practice. Attention to these matters quickly pays dividends in improved treatment, as would further research. Dean and Howell (1986), Greenberg, Kuczaj and Suppiger (1983), Hakes (1980) and Taylor (1982) have contributed to the exploration of this potentially fruitful area.

It will be realised that *metapragmatic* awareness and metapragmatic behaviour involve perceiving and acting upon the knowledge of factors which contribute to optimal communication; for instance remembering to face listeners who are hard of hearing and to include multiple cues when addressing them; simplifying language addressed to those with processing difficulties; noticing that communication failure has occurred and taking steps towards repair; sensing that failure is about to occur and attempting to prevent it or to encourage persistence. Here is an example of a linguist offering just such encouragement:

> One way of preventing panic and mental paralysis in the face of problems which have so far defeated linguists, sociologists and philosophers is to study in detail a particular transcript — it will provide some initial arguments that such conversational data are, after all, manageable — there will also be however brief glimpses into the theoretical chasms over which we are suspended (Stubbs, 1983, p. 15) — [quite so!]

Clearly metapragmatics constitutes the fundamental expertise of communication therapists and speech pathologists, though very little has been written about their professional skills from this viewpoint. Clearly, too, it is in this area that many of their clients have difficulty. Whether these difficulties arise for constitutional reasons or as a result of other deficits or external influences is not at all clear at present. This means that the planning of treatment has to depend partly upon personal belief. Research into the effects of various treatment approaches is long overdue, and should lead to more realistic accountability at a time when this is being demanded in a fairly uninformed way.

In conclusion it is hoped that, as speech and language clinicians become familiar with the pragmatics literature, and as further investigations of clinical interaction take place, attention in assessment and treatment will once again focus upon the personal and communicative needs of clients. In these circumstances it will be possible to build upon present knowledge of behavioural techniques, physiological mechanisms, cognitive processes and linguistic structures to provide an excellent service. Valid communicative strategies (Faerch and Kasper, 1983) need no longer be mistaken for errors and 'corrected' at the expense of interactive confidence, but neither will the clinician assume that tuition in the production and use of specific language structures is always unnecessary.

Linguists may realise that their presence in schools and clinics can be of considerable value, and may thereby gain access to material which is, in turn, valuable for their particular purposes.

ACKNOWLEDGEMENTS

My thanks are due to John Connolly for consistently supporting my intention to explore this topic, and to Pam Grunwell and Diane Gordon for reading and commenting on an earlier version of this chapter. Errors or misconceptions in the present version are my own.

REFERENCES

Austin, J. (1962) *How to do things with words*, Clarendon Press, Oxford

Baron-Cohen, S., Leslie, A.M. and Frith, U. (1985) Does the autistic child have a 'theory of mind'? *Cognition, 21*, 37-46

Bates, E. (1974) Acquisition of pragmatic competence. *Journal of Child Language, 1*, 277-81

Bates, E. (1976) *Language and context: the acquisition of pragmatics*, Academic Press, New York

Bates, E., Camaioni, L. and Volterra, V. (1975) The acquisition of performatives prior to speech. *Merrill-Palmer Quarterly, 21*(3), 205-26

Bloom, L. and Lahey, M. (1978) *Language development and language disorders*, John Wiley and Sons, New York

Bruner, J. (1975) The ontogenesis of speech acts. *Journal of Child Language, 2*, 1-19

Colmar, S. and Wheldall, K. (1985) Behavioural language teaching: using natural language environment. *Child Language Teaching and Therapy*, 1(2), 199-216

Connolly, J. (1986) Intelligibility: a linguistic view. *British Journal of Disorders of Communication, 21*(3), 371-6

Conti-Ramsden, G. and Gunn, M. (1986) The development of conversational disability: a case study. *British Journal of Disorders of Communication, 21*(3), 339-51

Coulthard, M. (1985) *An introduction to discourse analysis*, Longman, London

Davis, G. and Wilcox, M. (1981) Incorporating parameters of natural conversation in aphasia treatment. In R. Chapey (ed.), *Language intervention strategies in adult aphasia*, Williams and Wilkins, Baltimore

Dean, E. and Howell, J. (1986) Developing linguistic awareness: a theoretically based approach to language disorders. *British Journal of Disorders of Communication*, 21(2), 223-38

De Hart, G. and Maratsos, M. (1984) Children's acquisition of presuppositional usage. In R.L. Schiefelbusch and J. Pickar (eds), *The acquisition of communicative competence*, University Park Press, Baltimore

Dik, S. (1978) *Functional grammar*, North Holland, Amsterdam

Dore, J. (1974) Holophrases, speech acts and language universals. *Journal of Child Language*, 2, 21-40

Dore, J. (1979) Conversational acts and the acquisitions of language. In E. Ochs, and B. Schieffelin, (eds), *Developmental pragmatics*, Academic Press, New York

Edmondson, W. (1981) *Spoken discourse: a model for analysis*, Longman, New York

Faerch, C. and Kasper, G. (1983) *Strategies in interlanguage communication*, Longman, London

Fillmore, C.J. (1975) Santa Cruz Lectures on Deixis 1971; mimeo, Indiana University Linguistics Club

Gallagher, T.M. (1983) Pre-assessment: a procedure for accommodating language use variability. In T.M. Gallagher and C.A. Prutting (eds), *Pragmatic assessment and intervention issues in language*, College Hill Press, San Diego

Greenberg, J., Kuczaj II, S.A. and Suppiger, A.E. (1983) An examination of adapted communication in young children. *First Language*, 4, 31-40

Grice, H.P. (1975) Logic and conversation. In P. Cole, and J.L. Morgan (eds), *Syntax and semantics, vol. 3: Speech acts*, Academic Press, New York

Hakes, D.T. (1980) *The development of metalinguistic abilities in children*, Springer Verlag, Berlin

Halliday, M.A.K. (1975) *Learning how to mean*, Edward Arnold, London

Halliday, M.A.K. (1985) *An introduction to functional grammar*, Edward Arnold, London

Hart, G. (1986) Incidental strategies. In R.L. Schiefelbusch (ed.), *Language competence: assessment and intervention*, Taylor & Francis, London

Haynes, C. (1986) A description of school children with semantic and pragmatic problems. Semantic and Pragmatic disorders Colloquium. University of Newcastle-upon-Tyne, UK

Holland, A. (1980) *Communicative abilities in daily living*, University Park Press, Baltimore

Leonard, L. (1981) Facilitating linguistic skills in children with specific language impairment. *Applied Psycholinguistics*, 2(2), 89-118

Letts, C. (1985) Linguistic interaction in the clinic: how do therapists do therapy? *Child Language Teaching and Therapy*, 1(3), 321-31

Leudar, I, (1981) Strategic communication in mental retardation. In W.I. Fraser and R. Grieve (eds), *Communicating with normal and retarded children*, John Wright & Sons, Bristol

Levinson, S.C. (1983) *Pragmatics*, Cambridge University Press, Cambridge

Longacre, R.E. (1979) The paragraph as a grammatical unit. In T. Givon, (ed.), *Syntax and semantics*, vol. 12: *Discourse and syntax*, Academic Press, New York

Lucas, E.V. (1980) *Semantic and pragmatic language disorders: assessment and remediation*, Aspen Systems Corporation, Maryland

Maassen, B. (1986) The role of temporal structure and intonation in deaf speech. In C. Johns-Lewis (ed.), *Intonation in discourse*, Croom Helm, Beckenham

McTear, M. (1985a) *Children's conversation*, Blackwell, Oxford

McTear, M. (1985b) Pragmatic disorders: a question of direction. *British Journal of Disorders of Communication*, 20(2), 119-27

McTear, M. (1985c) Pragmatic disorders: a case study of conversational disability. *British Journal of Disorders of Communication*, 20(2), 129-42

Ochs, E. and Schieffelin, B.B. (1979) *Developmental pragmatics*, Academic Press, New York

Panagos, J.M., Bobkoff, K. and Scott, C.M. (1986) Discourse analysis of language intervention. *Child Language Teaching and Therapy*, 2, 211-29

Piaget, J. and Inhelder, B. (1969) *The psychology of the child*, Basic Books, New York

Prutting, C.A. (1982) Pragmatics as social competence. *Journal of Speech and Hearing Disorders*, 2, 123-34

Ratner, N. and Bruner, J. (1978) Games, social exchange and the acquisition of language. *Journal of Child Language*, 5, 391-402

Rice, M. (1984) Cognitive aspects of communicative development. In R.L. Schiefelbusch, and J. Pickar (eds), *The acquisition of communicative competence*, University Park Press, Baltimore

Ripich, D.N. and Panagos, J.M. (1985) Accessing children's knowledge of sociolinguistic rules for speech therapy lessons. *Journal of Speech and Hearing Disorders*, 50, 335-346

Ripich, D.N., Hambrecht, G. and Panagos, J.M. (1984) Discourse analysis and aphasia therapy. *Aphasia–Apraxia–Agnoxia*, 3, 9-18

Roulstone, S. (1981) Out of the broom cupboard. *Special Education, Forward Trends*, 10(1), 13-15

Sarno, M. (1969) *The functional communication profile: manual*, New York University Medical Centre, New York

Searle, J. (1969) *Speech acts*, Cambridge University Press, Cambridge

Searle, J. (1975) Indirect speech acts. In P. Cole, and J.L. Morgan (eds), *Syntax and semantics*, vol. 3: *Speech acts*, Academic Press, New York

Sinclair, J. and Coulthard, R.M. (1975) *Towards an analysis of discourse*, Oxford University Press, London

Smith, B.R. (1986) The application of linguistic theory to the work of speech therapists with special reference to pragmatics and discourse analysis. Conference paper, British Association for Applied Linguistics. Leicester Polytechnic, UK

Smith, B.R. (1987a) 'Management' an outdated concept. AFASIC International Symposium, Specific Speech and Language Disorders in Children, University of Reading, UK

Smith, B.R. (1987b) The cautious revolution. International Pragmatics Conference. University of Antwerp, Belgium

Snow, C.E. (1984) Parent–child interaction and the development of communicative ability. In R.L. Schiefelbusch and J. Pickar, (eds), *The acquisition of communicative competence*, University Park Press, Baltimore

Snow, C., Midkiff-Borunda, S., Small, A. and Proctor, A. (1984) Therapy as social interaction: analysing the context for language remediation. *Topics in Language Disorders*, 4(4), 72-85

Stott, D.H. (1966) *Studies of troublesome children*, Humanities Press, London

Strawson, P.F. (1964) Intention and convention in speech acts. *Philosophical Review*, *73*, 439-60

Stubbs, M. (1983) *Discourse analysis. The sociolinguistic analysis of natural language*, Basil Blackwell, Oxford

Taylor, M. (1982) Explicit models of language: a child's eye view of language functions. *First Language*, *3* 223-6

Tizard, B. and Hughes, M. (1984) *Young children learning, talking and thinking at home and at school*, Fontana, London

Tough, J. (1977) *The development of meaning*, Unwin Educational, London

Ulatawska, H.K., North, A.J. and Macaluso-Haynes, S. (1981) Production of narrative and procedural discourse in aphasia. *Brain and Language*, *13*, 345-71

Wardhaugh, R. (1985) *How conversation works*, Basil Blackwell, Oxford

Wells, G. (1981) *Learning through interaction: the study of language development*, Cambridge University Press, Cambridge

Wilcox, M. and Davis, G. (1982) A pragmatic model for aphasia treatment. *Journal of the Ohio Aphasiology Association*, *1*, 2-10

11

Language Dominance in Bilingual Children

Niklas Miller

Several official laws and directives (e.g. US Public Law 94-142, 1975; EEC Directive on the Education of Children of Migrant Workers 77/486/EEC) have, for various reasons, recognised that obliging children with limited proficiency in the language of a particular State to follow (all) their schooling through this language is unjust. Accordingly notions of mother-tongue teaching and educational programmes in language maintenance, enrichment and transfer have arisen, aimed at creating a less disadvantaged education for the child.

Implicit in these stipulations and recommendations is the idea that there is a dominant language; that one of a bilingual's languages is mastered better than the other. Implicit also is that this relationship can be somehow measured, that tests or procedures can be devised to carry out the measurement, and that having established the dominance configuration further (language development, intelligence, etc.), testing and instruction will be made more fair. It is also tacitly assumed, and current practice largely bears this out, that once the dominance relationship has been determined, the nature of the balance between the languages will remain so across time and across different contexts. It has now been acknowledged for some time (Gerken, 1978; DeBlassie, 1980) that it is important for teachers and therapists to pay attention to the dominance factor in decision making and policy planning in children's education. The question to be asked here, though, is whether current notions of dominance are justified on theoretical and practical grounds, and whether they are to the child's benefit or simply add to the disadvantages thrust upon the child by dubious means to suspect ends. This chapter aims to point out some theoretical objections to the view that a bilingual manifests dominance simply in one language or another, and to draw implications from this for assessment and teaching of bilingual children. Clearly all possible objections cannot be aired in this context. Most importantly, in focusing on psycho- and sociolinguistic factors there will be omission of the political and socio-economic determinants which must be seen as the ultimate facilitators or bars to progress in the area.

LANGUAGE USE IN BILINGUAL SETTINGS

A rider of the assumption that there exists a straightforward equation 'language A (L_A) is more dominant than language B (L_B)' or vice-versa, is the notion that, for whatever reason (because it was acquired first; because most people in the community speak it; because legislation demands it etc.), this dominance relationship remains constant, and is unchanging over time and place. The view also implies that the pattern of dominance will be equal for all aspects of language function; not only listening, speaking, reading and writing, but within these categories for their subcomponents — phonology, syntax, morphology, lexicon and semantics. Such a position has been commonly extended from the individual to apply to all bilinguals in an assumed speech community. Hence it is assumed that all Spanish–English bilinguals in North America, or all Irish–English bilinguals in Ireland, will present a comparative picture. The position to be argued here is that the profile of dominance is not constant but is dynamic and fluid, both over different situations and at both societal and individual levels over time. It is suggested that the grossly oversimplified perspective on the relationship between a bi- or multilingual's languages, however well motivated in terms of searching for an avenue of fair assessment, is both flawed and ultimately divisive.

Earlier notions of bilingualism looked towards the competent, ideal bilingual as one who had balanced, native-like control of both languages. Anything less than this was deemed unsatisfactory and undesirable. A period when control of the different languages was unequal might have been tolerated as a transitionary phase while the person brought up the second language to the standard of the first, or while the person 'progressed' (since such was the assumed desirable state) to being a competent monolingual person, usually in the language of the dominant cultural–political society. Grosjean (1985) has even spoken of this ethic, the legacy of which is still very much alive, as the monolingual or fractional view of bilingualism. According to the strong version of the view the only true bilingual is one at or approaching native-like competence in both languages. The bilingual is regarded as a bi-monolingual — two monolingual speakers in one person. By the same token any contact (switching, mixing, interference) between the two languages is considered as diluting or polluting the naturalness and integrity of the pure forms of the respective languages.

The consequence has been that study of bilinguals in educational and clinical fields has tended to concentrate on their languages as separate entities, both from the acquisition and usage points of view, and from the point of view of the effects of one language on the other. This has tended to be in terms of two independent languages in contact rather than the two (or more) languages functioning as an integrated whole. The clinical-educational by-products of the bi-monolingual line of thought have been that assessments have been conducted with reference to separate monolingual norms, in extreme cases completely ignoring one of the languages (invariably the so-called 'minority' language). Teaching of children not suffering from handicapping conditions (though for many bilingualism itself was seen as a handicap to be eradicated) was thought to be best directed at one language. Where periods of bilingual schooling were introduced this was done in the belief that it would ease or speed the transition towards monolingualism in one of the languages. Language work for children with true handicapping conditions similarly was thought to be ideally conducted in one (this usually meant the majority community) language.

A less strong version of the bi-monolingual view concedes that other states of bilingualism exist than balanced (near) native competence in two languages. It is acknowledged that there may be dominance (greater ability) in one language over the other. The apparent positive result this has for teaching and therapy is that before decisions are made as to which language a child should be tested or taught in, an attempt is made to ascertain which is the child's better language. However, the question remains, is the latter task a straightforward possibility?

Numerous methods have been adopted to accomplish a dominance measure — such as speed of reaction (e.g. to responding to commands) in the two languages, speed of translating from one to the other, ease of switching from one language to another, the degree of interference in one language from the other, and contrasting of scores on (assumed) comparable tests of vocabulary (James, 1974; Nelson-Burgess and Myerson, 1975) or syntax (Burt, Dulay and Hernández-Chávez, 1976) in the respective languages. Aside from the reliability of the measures themselves, the main objection to the validity of these tests is that the (bi-monolingual) view of bilingualism on which they rest is incompatible with actual bilingual behaviour.

Fishman (1968) long ago pointed out that in stable bilingual situations a community is unlikely to maintain two languages that perform exactly the same communicative functions. If that were the case one of them would be redundant and not be liable to be kept on. The normally found situation is that where two or more languages are spoken side by side there is a functional differentiation in their usage. One language is associated with particular persons, settings, styles and occasions, while the other is used in a *complementary* contrasting, not competing, set of circumstances. The result is that the languages are used for quite different purposes, and an individual's competence in either will be closely related to the nature and frequency of access to the situations in which the particular language is employed.

This contrasts starkly with the bi-monolingual idea of bilingual language use. There the languages are seen as more or less interchangeable, functioning largely independent of each other, the only difference being in degree of mastery which is seen basically in terms of how long/much the person has been exposed to L_A or L_B. The latter assumption is the rationale behind those bilingual 'remediation' programmes which concentrate essentially on compensating for shortfalls simply by affording the child increased or intense exposure to the non-dominant language.

In that view of bilingualism which considers the two (or more) languages as complementing each other and acting interdependently a different perspective on the dominance issue emerges. In this case the individual's language competence, or more broadly communicative competence, cannot be gauged by examination of one language alone. Each language individually covers only part of the person's linguistic repertoire. Formal registers, and all the lexico-syntactic factors this involves, may be associated with one language; informal ones with the other, or with a mixed code. Daily living activities (entertainment, family chat, local shopping, religious obligations) may be conducted in one language; work, schooling and wider administrative matters (dealing with teachers, health workers, municipal services) may be performed in the other. Apart from the human interactional, sociopolitical background to why the pattern of usage might be, the direct implications for language assessment and teaching are that each of the separate situations in which a language is used makes differing demands on lexicon, syntax, morphology and semantics. While the monolingual has access to the range of styles and structures in one language, the bilingual has these spread through two (and maybe a third mixed version) languages.

The consequences for the dominance argument and assessing language ability are clear. By focusing on one dimension of language (phonology; lexicon, etc.) one will derive a biased reading of a person's linguistic ability, since in each of the languages different demands will be made on the subsystem, and the nature of the communicative experience will dictate what aspects of the subsystem have been acquired and how they are used. This bias is not removed by assessing in the one language as a whole, since it too will be associated with only a portion of the person's linguistic and experiential repertoire. How to overcome this skewing factor is discussed below.

Hence in the holistic view of bilingualism a mixed pattern of dominance is found. A person might be dominant in the lexicon of one language but the syntax of the other. They may even show varying dominance of subaspects of one component. They may be dominant for the syntax involved in discussing scientific matters in L_A but have the syntactic ability, or agility, for telling jokes or stories only in L_B. Again there are clear implications for teaching. Children may be experiencing difficulty in the classroom because the pattern of usage experience assumed is different, not because they are overall less competent or non-dominant in a language. That is, they are being obliged to perform functions with a part of the language unfamiliar to them. Any extra assistance they might need should then not be with L_A or L_B as a whole, but with the subaspect of it which assessment should identify.

In as far as the bilinguals' languages function as a whole, fulfilling the same roles that a monolingual's single language does, the only way to gain a true picture of their language ability is to assess them permitting input and output in the same pattern as they would use in everyday life. This implies use of the preferred language when, where and with whom it would normally be spoken/read. It also implies accepting the occurrence of code switching and mixing. Implicit in the bi-monolingual approach is the view that mixed codes, or interlanguages, are somehow not proper languages, either because they represent impure versions of the respective base languages, or because they are considered transitional stages in acquiring or losing a language.

However, far from reflecting imperfect or transitional forms of L_A or L_B the use of mixed codes in bilingual settings is typically an integral part of the person's and community's language repertoire. It is true that sometimes elements of L_A appear in L_B because the speaker does not have the necessary part of L_B available, but even this strategy tends to be rule-governed. There are times and places when this strategy is acceptable, and situations when alternative communicative strategies would have to be employed. More widely, a complex set of rules governs when code mixing will occur, the nature and extent of it and the communicative implications of this. Miller (1984b) has argued that far from seeing language usage in bilingual communities as revolving around the discrete poles of L_A and L_B, it is more realistic to consider a person's/community's linguistic repertoire as ranging along a continuum where L_A and L_B (which might seldom be spoken in their monolingual purist form) are only opposite ends of a scale where each discrete point blends into the next.

In many communities, indeed, the centre ground of the continuum might become a main medium of communication. Instances would be Tex-Mex in the South-eastern USA, or Pidgin and Creole languages which are examples par excellence of such interlanguages. This highlights once more why it is erroneous to conceive that one can identify a dominant language in a child, and assess the child in relation to the norms of monolingual users of that language.

It also highlights another point. Just as monolingual speech communities vary in how they mark different registers and convey nuances of meaning, so do bilingual communities. It is a fallacy to think that one can apply the norms of one bilingual community to the next. While there may be commonalities, the emphasis speakers from different communities will put on different parts of the L_A–L_B continuum, and the reasons they will move along it, will vary. Irish–English bilinguals in Dublin who have acquired Irish as a school subject will demonstrate patterns different from Irish–English bilinguals in Donegal where Irish is still a live language, despite the indifference, bordering on neglect, of the central government. They in turn will have a usage contrasting with Irish–English bilinguals in Belfast where the attitudes, official and popular, to the respective languages and the implications of commitment to bilingualism are different yet again. Similarly one should not expect Spanish–English speakers in New York, Texas and California, nor Gujarati–English speakers in Leicester, Nairobi and India to form a homogeneous language community. The lessons for assessment are that not only should one design assessment and teaching tools that are tuned to the bilingual continuum as a linguistic whole, but one should also attend to local usage and local norms.

The perspective given of bilingualism, and the problem of establishing which language is dominant, has emphasised that the relationship of a person's languages one to another is not of a static once and for all nature. Rather the relationship is fluid and dynamic, varying from one aspect of the language system to another in accordance with a complex of sociolinguistic determiners. The question of change and variability in the interrelationship of L_A and L_B is not, however, dictated solely by sociolinguistic factors. Another source of fluidity, central to clinical and educational considerations, is the state of flux existing during the acquisition process.

Acquisition and dominance

The issue of acquisition processes poses many questions for dominance decisions. Old-fashioned notions accepted implicitly or explicitly that one language was dominant, either because it was acquired first, was associated with the home (which assumes the home was monolingual or reflected the same dominance pattern as the child), or was the language of instruction. Through this focus the variations deriving from the different patterns and contexts of bilingual acquisition were neglected. It is precisely these matters that are likely to concern those assessing language development, or placement/language

241

of instruction questions — i.e. deciding from the dynamism and variability, which are inherent to bilingual language acquisition, what is normal development and what features represent a departure from that expected.

For instance, earlier studies did not address the question of what differences there might be in acquisition and usage between children who learned their two (or more) languages side by side from the start (so-called simultaneous acquisition) and those where onset of learning was staggered (i.e. sequential acquisition). In the former no attention was paid to whether there was a stable relationship between who spoke L_A and who spoke L_B, nor to where it might be spoken. In the latter there was scant regard to whether L_2 acquisition was commenced prior to or after the onset of formal education. Neither was there any consideration of the fate of L_1 after L_2 onset, especially if the child was going to be obliged to follow instructions and eventually gain employment exclusively in L_2. At the most the study of the interaction of L_1 and L_2 extended to examination of how the formal structure facilitated or impeded the acquisition of L_2 formal features, and how L_2 errors could be predicted or explained (this is interference and error analysis theory).

This leads into another debate, which has only been seriously studied over the past few years. That is, what are the similarities and differences psycholinguistically between L_1 and L_2 acquisition. Is L_2 learnt through L_1; are they acquired largely independently but along the same lines as regards order of acquisition, processes involved, etc.; are they acquired both independently, and by different psycholinguisitic processes; are there differences according to whether the languages are learned in naturalistic settings or through formal instruction.

All these queries, and many more, are relevant to assessing bilingual children — whether it is in making descriptive developmental profiles, devising and norming formal tests or interpreting individual or overall linguistic behaviours. It is not possible in this brief chapter to examine all these issues and their relation to classroom or clinic practices. The issues have been laid out recently by Dulay, Burt and Krashen (1982), Kessler (1984), Ellis (1985); and Skinner (1985a,b) who attempted to draw various theoretical strands together to develop a model of analysis for examining the mutual interdependence of language, language proficiency and learning.

Some points from the acquisition literature that have bearing on the dominance issue can be mentioned.

Alongside views that see language acquisition as largely a matter of activating or learning a set of formal (underlying) language rules, there have always been those who maintain that the acquisition of lexical items and syntactic structures is only part of the story. In the recent past thinking in this direction has been most notably stimulated by Hymes's (1971, 1985) concept of communicative competence. As well as having the basic, age-expected syntactic structures at its disposal, (syntactic, grammatical competence) the child must also 'know' 'rules' for when and how it is appropriate to use these structures (sociolinguistic competence), how to structure, maintain and operate these towards their desired end in exchanges (discourse competence); and how to act when they realise their formal competence is letting them down (strategic competence).

Typically competence between and within these areas does not proceed in a uniform, parallel fashion. For various reasons (changing intensity of input of L_A, L_B ...; age of commencing acquisition, being two most prominent factors) there is unevenness of advancement. An obvious cause is that L_A is heard from all but a few people, and in all but a few circumstances. The balance here may change as the child is obliged to function in more L_B situations — e.g. on school entry or gaining friends outside the home. More subtle variations may occur as the degree and standard of input changes. During the long school holidays children who rely primarily on school contacts (teacher, peers) for input in a language may slow considerably, or reverse in acquisition of this language, altering the surface dominance pattern. The arrival in the home of someone (relatives from another area, lodgers) which necessitates a change in the home language use pattern may alter the balance of competence.

Though the role of formal instruction in determining the outcome and rate of acquisition (Long, 1983; Ellis, 1985) is disputed, this may alter the balance in certain areas of competence. Likewise, while there are claims for universal order of acquisition of certain formal features (Cook, 1985) order within the alleged stages may be influenced by the need to communicate about certain things (Yoshida, 1978), by the age of acquisition (Dulay *et al.*, 1982; Ellis, 1985), or differences in complexity of certain formal features (Hickey, 1985).

Different competencies might emerge at separate rates and

243

orders. One child could have relatively good grammatical competence (e.g. because of formal instruction), but not know how to use this appropriately (poor sociolinguistic competence), while another child might have good strategic and sociolinguistic competencies but poor grammatical competence. Of the two on formal language tests the former child is likely to emerge as better or more dominant in the particular language; but as an effective communicator the second child would more likely be dominant.

In the past sociolinguistic and strategic competence has not been emphasised as consequential in language acquisition. Showing evidence of acquisition of specified structures has been a more salient criterion. However, it is now recognised that competencies other than grammatical are potent facilitators of communicative competence. Good sociolinguistic competence will give a good access to other speakers and situations more than mere formal skill would. Strategic competence will enable the child to gain access to, and hold open, channels not open to another child who lacks these facilities. The child who already has these skills in L_1 is more likely to proceed successfully in L_2 than the child who does not possess them. It is precisely these pragmatic competencies that appear to be lacking in some language-disordered children.

The implications here, for the dominance debate, are that relative dominance in one competence (grammatical; sociolinguistic ...) will fluctuate over time in the one child and between children of the same speech community. Similarly an individual need not be (equally) dominant in all competencies. The picture gained will vary also according to how dominance is judged and what demands are being made on the speaker–hearer. A child might appear to have a balanced command between L_A and L_B until it comes to school work, which places different demands on the linguistic system. This stresses the importance of analysing the child's language systems as a whole, and not merely single dimensions of it in isolation. Many of the issues in dominance variability, dependent on which competencies are examined, when and how, relate to the debates over so-called semilingualism (Cummins, 1979; Skutnabb-Kangas, 1981; Edelsky, Altwerger, Barkin, Flores, Hudelson and Jilbert, 1983; Martin-Jones and Romaine, 1986) and threshold hypotheses (Cummins, 1977; Diaz, 1985). Unfortunately this line cannot be pursued here.

Some other points from the acquisition literature that have direct bearing on the dominance issue are also worth mentioning as challenges to the bi-monolingual view of language dominance.

A typical feature of simultaneous acquisition is code mixing. Such behaviour was formerly considered as evidence for incomplete mastery of the language(s) and as negative. Actual study of children learning simultaneously (see Kessler, 1984) has shown mixing to be a natural feature in the acquisition process. There are at least two sources.

Firstly the language input may be a mixed code. The extent to which this attains will be a function of the practices within the broader community and more narrowly in the family and peer circle of the infant. As was stressed above, in many bilingual communities what are perceived by the speakers to be stretches of L_A or L_B might be far from the monolingual forms of those languages, and be only in fact a minor shift from the centre point of the L_A–L_B continuum. Further, the actual varieties of L_A or L_B used within the (sub)community may well not be standard varieties. They may be examples of, or combinations of, local regional variations, lingua franca varieties typical of areas where there are groups of bilingual speakers who use one of the languages as a common denominator but have different other languages (e.g. English between Punjabi and Bengali speakers in London; Bavarian German between Turkish and Italian speakers in Munich), or interlanguage varieties if the parents are in the process of becoming bilingual (or monolingual).

Secondly from the individual's point of view when acquiring languages simultaneously, amongst the many divisions discernible, there exists a period before the child has achieved sufficient metalinguistic awareness to be able to separate the two languages, during which the resultant mixed-language develops along identical lines to any other single language. This is to say that acquisition proceeds through one-word holophrastic utterances, to two-word utterances, phrases with omission of certain auxiliary markers and so on. Not until around age two years, six months does a functional and acquisitional differentiation emerge. This latter follows a pattern determined by the usage within the child's language sphere. It is then that code switching as opposed to habitual mixing gradually comes to predominate.

Such a period of code mixing of a cognitive–linguistic origin is not as typical in sequential acquisition, and becomes less likely the greater the age at which L_2 is commenced. A different source of mixing in the sequential learner's case is the strategy of falling back on L_1 to fill gaps in L_2 needs. This strategy may involve overt use of L_1 lexical items, or less obvious resort to L_1 in terms of using L_2 lexicon but L_1 syntax or semantics. Not permitting a child to adopt the strategy in test performance which works for him/her in everyday life will put the child at a disadvantage.

There may also exist a contrast in relative dominance between competencies on account of the pressure to communicate. Given the time and opportunity to formulate utterances children may display their maximum (expressive) grammatical knowledge. However, put under pressure to communicate (e.g. because of the urgency of the situation; or the need to play the 'answer as fast as you can' obligation demanded in typical western test situations) the child may sacrifice grammatical accuracy and resort to earlier, more familiar and easily commanded grammatical forms, or shift emphasis to his or her more reliable sociolinguistic and strategic competence. Either way, a different impression of dominance will be given.

A frequently reported phenomenon (see Dulay *et al.*, 1982, for instance, for a summary) in sequential acquisition is a silent period during which the child produces no or very little L_2 expressive language, despite being able to comprehend well. It is believed this may be a phase during which children are consolidating knowledge of L_2 to enable them to go ahead and use it without resort to L_1 when the time comes. Pressure on them to communicate during this phase forces them to use L_1-based strategies to succeed. Erroneous conclusions regarding relative dominance are liable to be drawn if this behaviour is misinterpreted (making assumptions that the child knows no L_2) or mishandled (cornering the child into using L_1-influenced utterances).

A similar silence phenomenon has been reported whereby bilingual children apparently reject one of their languages. This typically occurs when the one language becomes socially less necessary or desirable (Itoh and Hatch, 1978).

All these points go to emphasise that acquisition is not an even process predictable in its fine details. It is open to influences from external and internal (affective; personality; cognitive–linguistic maturity at onset of acquisition, etc.) factors. If these all render redundant the bi-monolingual view of language dominance relationships, what alternative perspectives offer themselves for practical solution? This is now briefly turned to.

IMPLICATIONS FOR ASSESSMENT AND THE NOTION OF DOMINANCE

Several points have already been drawn out above concerning the shortcomings of the bi-monolingual view of bilingualism and the naivety of the assumption that there is a simple equation of dominance–non-dominance between a bilingual's languages. This section draws these and other points together to work towards deriving a more accurate, and hence educationally/ clinically more pertinent and reliable, description of the individual's language functioning.

What is one going to assess?

Though some theoretical linguists may still treat language as an abstract set of rules divorced from live speakers, it is now firmly established that for clinical/educational purposes one's approach to assessment and teaching must be rooted in actual usage, whatever the lessons from theoreticians might be.

Hence an accurate picture of a person's language ability will not be gained by assessing and generalising from one aspect (lexical; syntactic, etc.) of his/her language functioning. Sampling a broad range of formal linguistic functions (testing to see if the child 'knows', can manipulate, the formal 'rules' of a language's grammar) will not compensate for this. Firstly because a bilingual's formal repertoire will not necessarily be embodied in L_A or L_B separately; and secondly because formal competence is only one aspect of language functioning required in gaining full communicative competence in a language.

A more reliable estimation can be worked towards by designing techniques that tap formal knowledge over the full range of the L_A–L_B continuum used by the child, and that permit responses according to the child's habitual pattern of response, not according to a tester's monolingual assumptions on norms in L_A versus L_B individually.

Such techniques need to be derived from studies of formal acquisition patterns and processes for the languages involved, and equally pertinently for the language community concerned (see below). The latter applies because while one might be able to identify universal trends (Dulay *et al.*, 1982; Ellis, 1985) in order, route and rate of acquisition, what is actually performed with the formal aspects of the language is embedded in the functional rules of the micro- and macrolinguistic community. Therefore it is imperative to compare a child's relative strengths in executing the *functions* of language as well as mastering the *forms*, since competence in one does not necessarily follow from competence in the other. Also, the different uses to which the person needs to put the language will make differential demands on competence in the various areas.

Evaluation must then include measures of the children's sociolinguistic competence — i.e. the ability to use formal grammatical rules appropriately in accordance with the participants, setting, topic and so on, of the interaction; their discourse competence — i.e. ability to produce utterances and exchanges forming a meaningful whole; and their strategic competence — i.e. ability to recognise and repair through correction or compensation for the shortcomings of their formal competence. This applies equally to monolingual subjects, but in dealing with bilingual people the evaluation must take place in the context of their multicultural situation.

In turn this poses questions of *how* one is going to assess bilingual communicative competence, and the content of these methods. Spolsky (1985) stresses the need to achieve authenticity in the material and methods. He discusses the limits of language tests in getting beyond the 'playing the rules' game in formal tests, and even the limits of authentic seeming tasks. He views the solution to the impasses as coming only from long, patient and sympathetic observation by observers who care to help. Observation (as stressed by Prutting, 1983; Mattes and Omark, 1984; Miller, 1984b) needs to take place in a variety of contexts that are going to accurately reflect the child's breadth (or narrowness) of usage. It is no use restricting observations and assessment to the type of language spoken/written in the classroom, since this will be quite different from that used at home, in the playground, with different peers and with other adults.

Diaries and questionnaires (Teitelbaum, 1979; J. Miller, 1981) have been used to gain a profile of the patterns of usage. Here one has to guard against the bias of observer expectations. They tend to note either what they think they themselves would say in the situation, or what they think community norms would dictate, rather than what linguistically objectively was spoken.

Tannen (1984) has summarised the areas that might be attended to in analysing the pragmatics of cross-cultural communication — viz. knowing when to talk, what to say, how to pace and pause, how to listen, intonation, formulaicity (conventional idiomatic versus novel usage in a language), indirectness (how to infer and imply the unspoken) and coherence and cohesion.

Damico, Oller and Storey (1983), Oller (1983), Prutting (1983) and Mattes and Omark (1984) have considered the task of carrying out evaluations of what bilinguals can do with their languages.

Mattes and Omark (1984) underline the importance in diagnosing for true language disability (as opposed to low performance in one language on the basis of limited experience with it), of the need to observe whether a child is actually succeeding in communicating with the language, whether children are able to work their language, whether or not there is formal accuracy. Thus they look for whether the child can initiate and maintain exchanges, whether or not these exchanges achieve their goal, whether the child is able to use (or resort to) necessary non-verbal paralinguistic back-up. They observe what functions the child is able to perform with the language, such as requesting, informing, finding out, regulating others and so on. Observations such as these require that clinicians know what functions language plays in the child's culture(s), how these functions are realised, and what aspects and manner of their manipulation are age-appropriate within the community.

Damico et al. (1983) and Oller (1983) found that referrals for more detailed diagnosis for learning problems were more frequent and more accurate if teachers were trained to examine pragmatic functions rather than concentrate solely on surface structure formal grammatical accuracy. They looked out for children who in their languages evidenced disproportionate (begging the question of what constitutes proportionate) linguistic non-fluencies, repeated revisions which ended in children boxing themselves in syntactically, delayed responses, over-use of non-specific referring terms ('thing', 'stuff', 'this', 'that' without apparent antecedent referents), frequent inappropriate responses, poor topic maintenance and need for speakers to give multiple repetitions before the child comprehends.

Olshtain and Blum-Kulka (1985) also focus on ways of assessing for communicative competence in second language acquisition. They discuss the difficulties inherent in gathering reliable background ethnolinguistic data and replicating more experimental methods in the testing situation. Their solutions (role play; open-ended questionnaires on usage in specified situations; discourse completion tests) are more suited to the older more linguistically aware child, but adaptations could be envisaged for younger, suspected learning-disabled children.

Another point brought out above was the diversity of usage even between and within communities using the same languages. This has to be taken into consideration when devising and standardising assessments. Ideally assessments should rest on community-based norms. Many practitioners (Evard and Sabers, 1979; Miller, 1984b) have called for such an approach, and recent scholarship has been applied to devising such norms (Toronto and Merrill, 1983; Mattes and Omark, 1984). In forming local scales one has not only to follow the usual procedures in producing reliable and valid items and tests, but also attend to preliminary questions which will dictate the content and language(s) of the test.

For instance, what varieties of the languages do the children come into contact with. Just because they are assumed to speak Spanish and English it does not follow that introducing test elements in Castillian Spanish and (British; North American; Australian) standard English is going to enable one to arrive at a more accurate assessment. What is the nature of the subjects' contact with the respective languages in terms of volume, context and sources of input. What demands are or will be made on them in their various languages in terms of formal and functional requirements. What are the typical patterns of acquisition and usage within the community. Has acquisition proceeded through formal, informal or both channels. What are broader and narrower community attitudes to the languages involved. All these factors and more will have bearing on the content of tests, and patterns of administration and response. The aim will be to tap as near as possible which features go together to represent the community's view of efficient communicative competence within the framework of their languages seen as a functional whole.

Assessments will also need to acknowledge the dynamic aspects of language — both from the acquisition and from the usage point of view. Language acquisition is not a simple linear process whereby one block is added step-wise to another. Each new stage in the process brings a qualitatively differently organised system, continuously in flux. Coupled with the variation stemming from changes in sociolinguistic, affective and motivational determiners, this means that the relationship amongst the bilinguals' languages and subparts of them is seldom stable. The bi-monolingual view largely ignored this. A holistic approach must embrace it.

CONCLUSION

This chapter has argued against the notion of a straightforward either L_A or L_B dominance in bilinguals. It has aimed to show the incompatibility of the line of thought from which simple dominance equations are derived. It has not meant to be an exhaustive exposition of these arguments (see Skutnabb-Kangas, 1981 and Grosjean, 1985 for more detailed consideration) but has illustrated the shortcomings of a unidimensional dominance configuration from usage and acquisition studies. While the chapter has also drawn conclusions for the clinic and classroom from the holistic approach to bilingual behaviours it has not meant to provide a step-by-step manual on assessment. Rather the aim has been to signpost a direction and establish a rationale that will enable a just and accurate evaluation of bilinguals' language.

There are many theoretical issues with practical implications that have only been hinted at here, or not mentioned at all, but whose resolution will advance practice in the field of assessing bilingual communicative competence.

For instance, are there universals in what is acquired (in terms of syntactic structures, semantic relationships marked) and how language is used at different stages of acquisition as some have argued (see above). If this is true, are these universals specific enough and accessible enough to be able to be used in assessment of language development and actual language usage. Even if one can identify broad stages in acquisition, how comparable are substages within the broader bands, both between individuals in monolingual groups and between different languages. Could the identification of such commonalities be exploited in constructing assessments dealing in units which would make tests valid and reliable across languages. At present it appears that, while trends can be discerned, the absolute order is fragile and open to influence from communicative demands and intralanguage psycholinguistic factors, again stressing the necessity of conducting evaluation of language usage within a pragmatic framework, undivorced from live usage. The challenge is to establish developmental norms of usage, so that even if there is variability in proximity to adult norms for marking specified features, one can observe whether the child is able to signal age-appropriately a given feature. The question of dominance then is not centred (solely) around the presence or not of lexical items, syntactic structures or whatever, but what the child can do as a communicator. The work of Oller *et al.* above is recalled.

Another issue relevant to the dominance question, and which language to conduct assessment and therapy in, is the relationship in the acquisition process between a bilingual's languages. Are L_A and L_B both learned via the same processes, i.e. does L_B learning = L_A learning? Does this hold for sequential as well as simultaneous acquisition? If it does not, what is the nature of the influences of L_A on L_B and vice-versa. Is there such a thing as acquisition of language principles that, once established, can be applied to any language encountered; and are these accessible for the purpose of language teaching and therapy? What is transferable between languages, what is the route of learning and how can this be influenced? Currently there are no straightforward answers, but again resolution will have relevance to gauging progress in acquisition in both monolingual and mixed language speakers.

In the meantime one is faced with the problem of how to walk the tightrope between the usefulness of formal tests, which elicit data on specific formal features but lose sight of language as live, and pragmatic approaches which stress overall communicative effectiveness, but at the expense, some would say, of attention to individual formal features.

A most vital area not examined in this chapter, but pertinent to the dominance issue, is sociopsychological factors at work. Personality, affective, motivational, attitudinal variables all play directly or indirectly (from the family, community) on the individual's acquisition and usage patterns. The cultural bias inherent in the construction and administration of different test types (Miller, 1984c; Chen and Henning, 1985) was only briefly hinted at. Neither was it examined why, in the latter quarter of the twentieth century, there should have arisen a notion of mother-tongue teaching, dominance, and to what ends they are used.

REFERENCES

Burt, M., Dulay, H. and Hernández-Chávez, E. (1976) *Technical handbook: bilingual syntax measure*, Harcourt, New York
Chen, Z. and Henning, G. (1985) Linguistic and cultural bias in language proficiency tests. *Language Testing, 2*(2), 155-63
Cook, V. (1985) Universal grammar and second language learning, *Applied Linguistics, 6*(1), 2-18
Cummins, J. (1977) Cognitive factors associated with the attainment of intermediate levels of bilingual skills, *Modern Language Journal, 61*, 3-12
Cummins, J. (1979) Linguistic interdependence and the educational development of bilingual children, *Review of Educational Research, 49*, 222-51
Damico, J., Oller, J. and Storey, M. (1983) The diagnosis of language disorders in bilingual children: surface-oriented and pragmatic criteria, *Journal of Speech and Hearing Disorders, 48*, 385-94
De Blassie, R. (1980) *Testing Mexican American Youth*, Teaching Resources, Hingham, Mass.
Diaz, R. (1985) Bilingual cognitive development: addressing three gaps in current research, *Child Development, 56*, 1376-88
Dulay, H., Burt, M. and Krashen, S. (1982) *Language Two*, Oxford University Press, Oxford
Edelsky, C., Altwerger, B., Barkin, F., Flores, B., Hudelson, S. and Jilbert, K. (1983) Semilingualism and language deficit, *Applied Linguistics, 4*(1), 1-22
Ellis, R. (1985) *Understanding second language acquisition*, Oxford University Press, Oxford
Evard, B. and Sabers, D. (1979) Speech and language testing with distinct ethnic-racial groups. A survey of procedures for improving validity, *Journal of Speech and Hearing Disorders, 44*, 255-70
Fishman, J. (1968) Sociolinguistic perspective on the study of bilingualism, *Linguistics, 38*, 21-50
Gerken, K. (1978) Performance of Mexican American children on intelligence tests. *Exceptional Child, 44*(6), 438-43
Grosjean, F. (1985) The bilingual as a competent but specific speaker–hearer, *Journal of Multilingual and Multicultural Development, 6*(6), 467-77
Hickey, T. (1985) Pronoun development in Irish. In P. Fletcher and M. Garman (eds), *Child language seminar papers*, University of Reading, UK
Hymes, D. (1971) *On communicative competence*, University of Pennsylvania Press, Philadelphia

Hymes, D. (1985) Toward linguistic competence, *AILA Review*, 2, 9-23

Itoh, H. and Hatch, E. (1978) Second language acquisition: a case study. In E. Hatch (ed.), *Second language acquisition*, Newbury House, Rowley, Mass.

James, P. (1974) *James language dominance test*, Teaching Resources, Hingham, Mass.

Kessler, C. (1984) Language acquisition in bilingual children. In N. Miller (1984a)

Long, M. (1983) Does second language instruction make a difference? *TESOL Quarterly*, *17*(3), 359-82

Martin-Jones, M. and Romaine, S. (1986) Semilingualism: a half-baked theory of communicative competence. *Applied Linguistics*, 7(1), 26-38

Mattes, L. and Omark, D. (1984) *Speech and language assessment for the bilingual handicapped*, College Hill, San Diego

Miller, J. (1981) *Assessing language production in children, experimental procedures*, Edward Arnold, London

Miller, N. (ed.) (1984a) *Bilingualism and language disability — assessment and remediation*, Croom Helm, London/College-Hill Press, San Diego

Miller, N. (1984b) Language use in bilingual communities. In Miller (1984a)

Miller, N. (1984c) Some observations regarding formal tests in cross-cultural settings. In N. Miller (1984a)

Nelson-Burgess, S. and Myerson, J. (1975) MIRA: a concept in receptive language assessment of bilingual children, *Language, Speech, Hearing Services in the Schools*, *6*, 24-8

Oller, J. (1983) Testing proficiencies and diagnosing language disorders in bilingual children. In D. Omark and J. Erickson (1983)

Olshtain, E. and Blum-Kulka, S. (1985) Cross-cultural pragmatics and the testing of communicative competence. *Language Testing*, *2*(1) 16-30

Omark, D. and Erickson, J. (eds) (1983) *The bilingual exceptional child*, College Hill, San Diego

Prutting, C. (1983) Assessing communicative behaviour using a language sample. In D. Omark and J. Erickson (1983)

Skinner, D. (1985a) Access to meaning: the anatomy of the language/learning connection. Part I. *Journal of Multilingual Multicultural Development*, *6*(2), 97-116

Skinner, D. (1985b) Access to meaning. Part II. *Journal of Multilingual Multicultural Development*, *6*(5), 369-88

Skutnabb-Kangas, T. (1981) *Bilingualism or not: the education of minorities*, Multilingual Matters, Clevedon

Spolsky, B. (1985) The limits of authenticity in language testing, *Language Testing*, *2*(1), 31

Tannen, D. (1984) The pragmatics of cross-cultural communication, *Applied Linguistics*, *5*(3), 189-95

Teitelbaum, H. (1979) Unreliability of language background self-rating of young bilingual children, *Child Study Journal*, *9*(1), 51-9

Toronto, A. and Merrill, S. (1983) Developing local normed assessment instruments. In D. Omark and J. Erickson (1983)

Yoshida, M. (1978) The acquisition of English vocabulary by a Japanese speaking child. In E. Hatch (ed.), *Second language acquisition*, Newbury House, Rowley, Mass.

Author Index

Subject Index